Invitation to Holistic Health

A Guide to Living a Balanced Life

Second Edition

Charlotte Eliopoulos, RN, MPH, PhD

Executive Director
American Association for Long Term Care Nursing

JONES AND BARTLETT PUBLISHERS
Sudbury, Massachusetts
BOSTON   TORONTO   LONDON   SINGAPORE

World Headquarters
Jones and Bartlett Publishers
40 Tall Pine Drive
Sudbury, MA 01776
978-443-5000
info@jbpub.com
www.jbpub.com

Jones and Bartlett Publishers
Canada
6339 Ormindale Way
Mississauga, Ontario L5V 1J2
Canada

Jones and Bartlett Publishers
International
Barb House, Barb Mews
London W6 7PA
United Kingdom

Jones and Bartlett's books and products are available through most bookstores and online booksellers. To contact Jones and Bartlett Publishers directly, call 800-832-0034, fax 978-443-8000, or visit our website www.jbpub.com.

Substantial discounts on bulk quantities of Jones and Bartlett's publications are available to corporations, professional associations, and other qualified organizations. For details and specific discount information, contact the special sales department at Jones and Bartlett via the above contact information or send an email to specialsales@jbpub.com.

The authors, editor, and publisher have made every effort to provide accurate information. However, they are not responsible for errors, omissions, or for any outcomes related to the use of the contents of this book and take no responsibility for the use of the products and procedures described. Treatments and side effects described in this book may not be applicable to all people; likewise, some people may require a dose or experience a side effect that is not described herein. Drugs and medical devices are discussed that may have limited availability controlled by the Food and Drug Administration (FDA) for use only in a research study or clinical trial. Research, clinical practice, and government regulations often change the accepted standard in this field. When consideration is being given to use of any drug in the clinical setting, the health care provider or reader is responsible for determining FDA status of the drug, reading the package insert, and reviewing prescribing information for the most up-to-date recommendations on dose, precautions, and contraindications, and determining the appropriate usage for the product. This is especially important in the case of drugs that are new or seldom used.

Production Credits
Publisher: Kevin Sullivan
Acquisitions Editor: Emily Ekle
Acquisitions Editor: Amy Sibley
Associate Editor: Patricia Donnelly
Editorial Assistant: Rachel Shuster
Production Assistant: Roya Millard
Marketing Manager: Rebecca Wasley
V.P., Manufacturing and Inventory Control: Therese Connell
Composition: Publishers' Design and Production Services, Inc.
Cover Design: Scott Moden
Cover Image: © kd/ShutterStock, Inc.
Printing and Binding: Malloy, Inc.
Cover Printing: Malloy, Inc.

Library of Congress Cataloging-in-Publication Data
Eliopoulos, Charlotte.
    Invitation to holistic health : a guide to living a balanced life / Charlotte Eliopoulos. — 2nd ed.
      p. cm.
    ISBN 978-0-7637-6112-7 (pbk.)
    1. Holistic medicine.   2. Medicine, Chinese.   I. Title.
    R733.E425 2010
    613—dc22
                                                                          2008050239

6048

Printed in the United States of America
13 12 11   10 9 8 7 6 5 4 3

Table of Contents

Acknowledgments

Appreciation is given to the following individuals who contributed to the first edition of this book.

1. Assessing Your Health Habits
   Anneke Young, RN, BSN, CNAT
   Nurse Amma Therapist
   Former Dean of School for Wholistic Nursing at New York College

2. Healthful Nutrition
   Ann McKay, RNC, MA, DI Hom, HNC
   Health and Wellness Consultant

3. Dietary Supplements
   Ann McKay, RNC, MA, DI Hom, HNC

4. Exercise: Mindfulness in Movement
   Barbara Ann Stark, MSN, FNP, HNC
   Faculty, Western Michigan University, Kalamazoo

5. Immune Enhancement: Mind/Body Considerations
   Barbara Ann Stark, MSN, FNP, HN
   Faculty, Western Michigan University, Kalamazoo

6. Flowing with the Reality of Stress
   Linda S. Weaver, RN, MSN, CCRN
   Clinical and Extended Studies Faculty
   Beth El College of Nursing

7. Growing Healthy Relationships
   Irene Wade Belcher, RN, MSN, CNS, CNMT, HNC
   Holistic Nursing Consultants

8. Survival Skills for Families
   Joyce Murphy, RN, BS, MSN, HNC
   The Northwood Nurse, Holistic Nurse Consultant

9. The Spiritual Connection
   Carole Ann Drick, RN, DNS, TNS, CP
   Founder, Conscious Awareness Inc

10. Balancing Work and Life
    Genevieve Bartol, RD, EdD, HNC
    Professor Emeritus, University of North Carolina, Greensboro

11. Creative Financial Health
    Marilee Tolen, RN, CHTP/I, HNC
    President, Marilee Tolen, Inc.

12. Environmental Effects on the Immune System
    Natalie Pavlovich, RN, PhD, DiHt, CNHP
    Professor, Duquesne University School of Nursing

13. Promoting a Healing Environment
    Katherine Young, RN, MSN
    Founder, Essentials of Life

14. The Power of Touch
    Charlene Christiano, RN, MSN, CS, ARNP, CHTP
    Adult Nurse Practitioner

15. Taking Life Lightly: Humor, the Great Alternative
    Julia Balzer Riley, RN, MN, HNC
    President, Constant Source Seminars
    Adjunct Faculty, University of Tampa

16. Understanding the Hidden Meaning of Symptoms
    Marsha McGovern, RN, MSN, FNP, CS
    Assistant Professor of Nursing, Kings College

17. Working in Partnership with Your Health Practitioner
    Marie Fasano Ramos, RN, MN, MA, CMT
    Holistic Nurse

18. Menopause: Time of the Wise Woman
    Cynthia Aspromonte, RNC, NP, HTP-I, HNC
    Nurse Practitioner, Holistic Women's Healthcare

19. Addictions: Diseases of Fear, Shame, and Guilt
    Joan Efinger, RN, CS, MA, MSN, DNSc, HNC
    Holistic Healing Research Consultant
    Nancy Maldonado, MA, PhD
    Consultant

Resources

Myra Darwish, RN, MSN, CS, HNC
Clinical Coordinator of Geropsychiatric Services
St. Mary's Medical Center
Palm Beach Community College

Preface

When the first edition of *Invitation to Holistic Health* was published in 2004, the impact of Americans' growing interest in being active, proactive participants in their health care was being significantly felt. Consumers were replacing the "blind obedience" relationship with their healthcare providers with that of a partnership in which they had a strong voice in directing their healthcare. The Internet allowed easy access to a wide range of new medical advancements and alternative and complementary therapies that once were known only in remote parts of the world. Conventional healthcare providers found that many consumers came to their office visits equipped with literature searches and information on therapies that were outside those typically used in conventional medicine. Furthermore, consumers were exposed to insights into the interrelationship and interdependency of the body, mind, and spirit; they came to appreciate that one's health needed to be viewed from a holistic perspective. The idea for this book was born against this backdrop.

The Meaning of Holism

It may be beneficial to define what is meant by holistic health before going any farther. The term holism refers to a whole that is greater than the sum of its parts. In other words, 1 + 1 + 1 = 3 or 5 or more. When applied to health, holism implies that the health and harmony of the body, mind, and spirit create a higher, richer state of health than would be achieved with attention to just one part, such as physical functioning. Although some people equate it with the use of complementary and alternative therapies, holistic health is a philosophy of care in which a wide range of approaches are used to establish and maintain balance within an individual. Complementary and alternative therapies may be part of the approach to holistic health promotion, but so can healthy lifestyle choices, counseling, prayer, conventional (Western) medical treatments, and other interventions.

The Holistic Model Versus the Medical Model

Few people would argue that holistic health makes good sense; however, to appreciate why the holistic model has been slow to implement, it is useful to understand a little about Western medicine, or the U.S. healthcare system. Actually, health care is a misnomer, as Western medicine has functioned under a sick care model that we have come to know as the biomedical model. The biomedical model was built on certain tenets, highly valued by scientific minds, that include the following:

- *Mechanism:* This belief advanced the concept that the human body is much like a machine, explainable in terms of physics and chemistry. Health is determined by physical structure and function, and disease is a malfunction of the physical part. Malfunctions and malformations are undesirable. Disease is treated by repairing the malformed or malfunctioning organ or system with physical or chemical interventions (e.g., drugs, surgery). Nonphysical influences on health status are not considered, and healing, dysfunction, and deformity serve no purpose.

- *Materialism:* This thinking considers the human body and its state of health as being influenced only by what is seen and measurable. Physical malfunction is the cause of illness; therefore, illness is addressed by concrete treatments. Emotional and spiritual states have no impact on health and healing.

- *Reductionism:* This thinking reduces the human body to isolated parts rather than a unified whole. Treatment of a health condition focuses on the individual organ or system rather than the whole being. Good health is judged as having body systems that function well, despite one's feelings or spiritual state.

The first major challenge to the biomedical model occurred in the 1960s when the relationship of body and mind began to be discussed. In retrospect, it is difficult to believe that the medical community was skeptical that the mind could cause illness, yet the resistance to accepting the body–mind connection was real. Similarly, recognition of the role of the spirit in the cause and treatment of illness has met similar skepticism. As the dust settles, however, healthcare practitioners are understanding the profound, dynamic relationship of body, mind, and spirit to health and healing and moving toward a holistic model of health care.

About This Book

This book offers guidance to you in your journey to holistic health. There are no special formulas provided that guarantee eternal youth and freedom from illness. There is no revolutionary diet or plan that will change your life in 30 days or less, and there are no exotic substances that you can use to develop a new you will be found among the pages of this book. Instead, solid principles for building a strong foundation for optimal health are presented with practical advice that you can easily adopt and integrate into your life.

The book is divided into three parts. In the first part, Strengthening Your Inner Resources, practices are discussed that can build your body's reserves and help it to function optimally. You will be guided through a self-assessment of your health habits so that you can determine areas that may need special attention. The realities of good nutrition are examined along with an in-depth look at dietary supplements. Exercise is approached from a body, mind, spirit perspective. Likewise, the important activity of enhancing your immune system is considered from a mind–body framework. Methods to flow with the inescapable reality of stress are discussed.

Developing Healthy Lifestyle Practices is the theme of the second part of this book. The many complex factors that influence your health status as you interact with the world beyond your body are addressed in chapters on topics such as growing healthy relationships, family survival skills, spirituality, humor, touch, and the environment. Recognizing the significant impact of work and money on one's total being, chapters are dedicated to each of these topics.

The third part of this book, Taking Charge of Challenges to the Body, Mind, and Spirit, offers information to equip you to be proactive in keeping yourself in balance. The hidden meaning of symptoms is explored to help you learn about the factors behind your health conditions. Practical advice is offered on how you can work in partnership with your healthcare provider to assure you get the best care possible. Transitions associated with menopause are examined, along with a wide range of approaches to manage the symptoms that may be experienced. Interesting insights into gambling, drugs, overeating, and other addictions are shared. With the growing use of complementary therapies, a chapter describing their purpose, benefits, and related precautions provides valuable information for sensible use of these products and practices. In addition, chapters focusing on herbs, aromatherapy, and homeopathic remedies offer practical insights into these popular therapies. Skills for being an effective caregiver are presented, along with a chapter outlining resources that can aid you in being an informed healthcare consumer.

This new edition of *Invitation to Holistic Health* provides the same basic chapters as the earlier edition. Information has been updated throughout. Significantly, current research on the effectiveness and safety of herbs and other complementary and alternative therapies has been incorporated, thereby causing some content changes in the "Safe Use of Complementary Therapies" and "Herbal Remedies" chapters. "Menopause: Time of the Wise Woman" was revised to reflect current thinking about the safe use of estrogen replacement, soy products, and other approaches to manage symptoms. Updates and additions have been included in other chapters as well. New suggested readings and resources have been provided for further exploration into topics.

A useful approach to using this book is to give it an initial fast read from cover to cover. This can be followed by a focus on chapters that address specific interests and needs. Although some of the chapters may not pertain to you directly (for instance, if you are not a caregiver you may not have a keen interest in "Surviving Caregiving"), you may find that a quick review of the chapter could acquaint you with its content so that you will recall it in the future if you or people who know are faced with this issue. You will probably find that the rich facts and resources provided make this book a great reference for your personal library.

Part I

Strengthening Your Inner Resources

Chapter 1

Assessing Your Health Habits

OBJECTIVES

This chapter should enable you to

- List at least six features of an ideal health profile
- Describe at least four questions that need to be considered in evaluating nutritional status
- Identify at least eight major areas to consider when taking stock of stress patterns
- Describe four areas involved in acquiring relaxation skills

Self-care is a term that is used to describe the active role people take in maintaining or improving their health. It is an aspect of health that is often overlooked when health care is discussed. Even in the arena of preventive medicine, which aligns the closest to the idea of self-care in modern medicine, the emphasis is more on the early detection of disease than the active promotion of health. Although there is a focus on health screening, less attention is given to educating people about healthy living habits, such as exercise, stress management, and nutrition.

Making minor adjustments in health practices to prevent diseases is easier than caring for diseases after they have developed. Prevention starts with taking stock of health habits and comparing them with those consistent with optimum health. By confronting the

---

KEY POINT

Americans have come to accept the World Health Organization's definition of health as a state of physical and mental well-being and not just the absence of disease; however, in traditional Chinese medicine (TCM), health is seen as the sufficient amount of energy circulating freely in the organism. TCM believes that the human being is comprised of and surrounded by an energy system or field. This energy system is understood to resemble an electromagnetic field, expressed on the minute level as the behavior of electrons and neurons and on the gross level as the experience of vitality. The energy system is made up of energy pathways, often referred to as meridians. The pathways are believed to carry energy and information throughout the human organism to unite body, mind, and spirit.

behaviors that lead to poor health, individuals can identify unhealthy practices and sources of imbalance and begin taking steps to change.

Basic Human Needs

To maintain a healthy state, people need to assure they are meeting basic human needs, which include the following:

- Respiration
- Circulation
- Nutrition
- Hydration
- Elimination
- Rest
- Movement
- Comfort
- Safety
- Connection with significant others, culture, the environment
- Purpose

Although these needs appear straightforward and simple, their fulfillment depends on some complex factors, such as physical, mental, and socioeconomic capabilities; knowledge, experience, and skill; and the desire and decision to take action.

Exploring the factors that impact the basic need for nutrition demonstrates the complexities at play. To maintain a healthy nutritional state, an individual needs to do the following:

- Know what constitutes a healthy diet
- Have the cognitive ability to plan, prepare, and consume meals
- Have the money to purchase food
- Be physically able to shop for, handle, prepare, and consume food
- Know how to cook
- Be motivated to eat properly
- Have an emotional state that is conducive to proper food intake
- Make sound dietary choices
- Organize activities to have the time to eat

When deviations from health are identified, it is useful to consider what factors could be contributing to the problem so that appropriate plans of correction can be developed.

For example, someone with an obesity problem who eats too much of the wrong foods may do so because he or she is depressed. Although classes that review healthy foods could be beneficial, behavioral changes may be more likely to occur if the person receives counseling and other treatment for depression.

Self-Assessment

An overall evaluation of health begins with a review of the current health status and health practices. An ideal health profile is one in which an individual

- Consumes an appropriate amount of quality food
- Exercises regularly
- Maintains weight within an ideal range
- Has effective stress coping mechanisms
- Balances work and play
- Looks forward to activities with energy and enthusiasm
- Falls asleep easily and sleeps well
- Eliminates waste with ease
- Has meaningful relationships
- Enjoys a satisfying sex life
- Feels a sense of purpose
- Is free from pain and other symptoms

When the ideal is not being met, there needs to be an exploration into the reasons so that strategies to improve health habits can be identified and implemented.

Physical Self-Assessment

Nutrition

In order to assess how nutritional habits impact health, a person's eating habits need to be evaluated for a period of time. Factors to consider include not just the type of foods consumed, but also the following:

- *When food is consumed:* Late-night eating puts extra stress on the digestive system. According to TCM, at night, the Yin (which is associated with rest, darkness, and stillness) predominates, and consequently, the digestive system slows down. The circulation slows down as well, conserving the amount of blood circulating to all of the digestive organs. Clearly, nighttime—when the body is supposed to be resting and preparing for restoring and repairing tissues—is not a good time to offer the body the challenge of digesting a big meal. Viewed from within the context of TCM, this behavior can lead to a condition called Stomach Yin Deficiency, which is a condition in which the fluids of the stomach diminish, causing a sensation of heat in the stomach, manifesting as heartburn and indigestion. When this condition is allowed to persist, more serious stomach problems, such as a hiatal hernia or ulcer may develop.

KEY POINT

Late night eating stresses the digestive system.

- *What one does while eating:* When there is emotional tension while eating, energy is diverted and less available for digestion. When stressed by heated conversations or upsetting news on the television, a person's energy is drawn away from the digestive system, causing indigestion. For optimum digestion adequate supplies of enzymes, co-enzymes, and hormones are needed, and in order for these substances to be available, adequate amounts of blood must be circulating. Free-flowing energy, or Qi, promotes blood flow. This emphasizes the importance of relaxing during mealtime so that there will be sufficient resources for digestion.

KEY POINT

In Traditional Chinese Medicine, Qi is considered the vital life force or energy that circulates throughout the body.

- *The amount that is consumed:* When too much food is consumed during a meal, the stomach gets stressed. This kind of behavior not only leads to indigestion, but also creates an energy deficit as energy is pulled from other areas to meet the demands of digestion. Between-meal nibbling creates the same kind of energy deficit, as energy is constantly required by the digestive organs to digest and not enough energy is available for other activities. Each time food is being consumed, blood is routed to the digestive organs, and less is available for other physiological activities, creating an imbalance in the body. In addition, the many muscle layers of the stomach need to rest for a certain amount of time.

REFLECTION

Consider what, when, and how you eat. Is your pattern conducive to having optimal energy available for other activities?

Identifying Patterns

Daily food journals that record food consumed, when it is consumed, and how one feels during food consumption can be beneficial in identifying patterns. Everything that enters the mouth—whether it is a piece of candy or a few sips of juice—should be recorded. Keeping this type of food diary increases self-awareness, which in turn can become the catalyst for positive changes in nutritional habits. After keeping a food journal for a couple of weeks, sufficient data will be available to determine the pattern and content of nutritional habits. Are meals being eaten on a regular basis? How much snacking is taking place? Are the foods chosen basically nutritious? Is one kind of food eaten in excess? Are some nutrients missing from the diet?

A review of beverage consumption is useful. What kinds of beverages are consumed? Is caffeine consumed from coffee and carbonated beverages, and if so, how much? Carbonated beverages are high in sugar or artificial sweetener, neither of which has any nutritional value. Caffeine is addictive, a mild stimulant to the central nervous system, and is a diuretic (fluid loss through urine). Mixed scientific reports exist about the role caffeine plays in health and wellness. Because caffeine affects many body systems and can interfere with certain drugs, it is best taken in moderation—no more than one or two cups of caffeinated beverages per day.

Alcoholic beverage intake needs to be captured, as well. What is the alcohol intake on an average day? Alcohol supplies no nutrients, but it does supply calories. High levels of alcohol intake increase the risk of stroke, heart disease, certain cancers, high blood pressure, birth defects, and accidents. Women should drink no more than one alcoholic beverage per day, and men should drink no more than two alcoholic beverages per day.

An evaluation of body weight is important, with attention to possible gradual increases in weight that may have been experienced with age. Maintaining weight within an ideal range is important to general health. Obesity has been on the rise for the last two decades, and approximately 30% of the adult population is obese. Obesity increases the risk of hypertension; heart disease; diabetes; arthritis; and uterine, breast, colon, and gall bladder cancers. People should be taught to use a weight chart to learn where their weight is in respect to their height (see Figure 1-1). The higher the weight for a specific height, the greater is the risk of health problems. Obese individuals need to be encouraged and assisted in implementing a reduction program; at minimum, they should commit to not gain any additional weight. On the other hand, being underweight for height or having a recent unexplained weight loss may be a sign of other health problems and warrants further diagnostic evaluation.

A deeper understanding of nutritional patterns and habits can be done by examining a person's childhood relationship with food. What were his or her habits and patterns of nutrition and diet during childhood? Does the individual continue to carry these patterns and habits? How does the childhood experience with food and eating affect current nutritional choices and lifestyle?

Figure 1-1   Body Mass Index (BMI) Table

BMI	19	20	21	22	23	24	25	26	27	28	29	30	31	32	33	34	35
Height	Weight (in pounds)																
4'10" (58")	91	96	100	105	110	115	119	124	129	134	138	143	148	153	158	162	167
4'11" (59")	94	99	104	109	114	119	124	128	133	138	143	148	153	158	163	168	173
5' (60")	97	102	107	112	118	123	128	133	138	143	148	153	158	163	168	174	179
5'1" (61")	100	106	111	116	122	127	132	137	143	148	153	158	164	169	174	180	185
5'2" (62")	104	109	115	120	126	131	136	142	147	153	158	164	169	175	180	186	191
5'3" (63")	107	113	118	124	130	135	141	146	152	158	163	169	175	180	186	191	197
5'4" (64")	110	116	122	128	134	140	145	151	157	163	169	174	180	186	192	197	204
5'5" (65")	114	120	126	132	138	144	150	156	162	168	174	180	186	192	198	204	210
5'6" (66")	118	124	130	136	142	148	155	161	167	173	179	186	192	198	204	210	216
5'7" (67")	121	127	134	140	146	153	159	166	172	178	185	191	198	204	211	217	223
5'8" (68")	125	131	138	144	151	158	164	171	177	184	190	197	203	210	216	223	230
5'9" (69")	128	135	142	149	155	162	169	176	182	189	196	203	209	216	223	230	236
5'10" (70")	132	139	146	153	160	167	174	181	188	195	202	209	216	222	229	236	243
5'11" (71")	136	143	150	157	165	172	179	186	193	200	208	215	222	229	236	243	250
6' (72")	140	147	154	162	169	177	184	191	199	206	213	221	228	235	242	250	258
6'1" (73")	144	151	159	166	174	182	189	197	204	212	219	227	235	242	250	257	265
6'2" (74")	148	155	163	171	179	186	194	202	210	218	225	233	241	249	256	264	272
6'3" (75")	152	160	168	176	184	192	200	208	216	224	232	240	248	256	264	272	279

Directions: Find your height in the left column. Go across the row to find your weight. Go up the column to the top row to find your BMI. Healthy BMI = 18–24.99. Overweight BMI = 25–29.99. Unhealthy BMI ("obese") = 30+.

Source: NIH/National Heart, Lung, and Blood Institute (NHLBI).

REFLECTION

Do you believe that if you make sensible nutrition choices you will live a healthier, more energetic life and reduce your risk of disease? Do you think that you can deviate from sound nutritional habits without consequences? What has influenced your beliefs? If your beliefs do not support good nutritional habits, what can you do to change them?

Often, small actions are all that are needed to realize significant change. This can be explored by evaluating the way lifestyle impacts eating habits, food preferences, and food choices. A short nutritional self-assessment (see Table 1-1) can assist with this effort. Approximately 10–15 minutes will be needed to complete the questionnaire. Writing the answers is important so that there will be a baseline to use for comparison after changes

TABLE 1-1 Nutritional Self-Assessment

· How would you rate your general health status?

· What is your height and weight? Are they within normal limits? Have there been any recent changes in height or weight?

· What health conditions do you presently have?

· Do you have any problems with your blood sugar? Elevated cholesterol or triglyceride levels? High blood pressure? Osteoporosis? Irritable bowel syndrome?

· Are you aware of any food intolerances or allergies?

· Do you consume adequate amounts of protein, fruits, and vegetables?

· Do you limit your intake of saturated fats and simple carbohydrates?

· Are you taking nutritional supplements, and if so, which ones?

· What is your pattern of eating? How many meals do you eat per day? What is the size of those meals?

· Do you snack regularly throughout the day or evening? During the night?

· How many snacks do you have per day? Of what do they consist?

· What is your energy pattern? Do you have any slumps during the day?

· How much caffeine through coffee, tea, and carbonated drinks do you drink per day?

· What is your alcohol intake?

· What is your coping style when under stress? Do you consume unhealthy foods or large quantities of food when you are feeling stressed, depressed, anxious, or unhappy?

· Do you tend to make healthy food choices?

have been made. The answers will help in determining whether there are nutritional imbalances (excesses or deficiencies). Decisions can then be made as to which foods need to be added and/or removed from the daily diet to improve nutrition.

The next step is to begin the process of eliminating or replacing foods that contribute to poor health. The intake of foods that are laden with artificial colorings, sweeteners, and preservatives should be reduced by half for the first few weeks and eventually eliminated altogether. Other foods that lead to ill health when consumed in excess are foods high in fat, refined sugar, salt, and dairy products.

KEY POINT

Paying attention to diet and nutritional habits does not mean that people need to become obsessed with eating to the point that they become stressed when they have an occasional slip from healthy eating. This stress could create an emotional imbalance, which has a negative effect on general health.

Fat

Eating high-fat foods such as ice cream, sour cream, cream cheese, hard cheese, heavy butter sauces, red meat, pork, duck, oil, and whole milk is a contributing factor in conditions such as atherosclerosis, heart disease, and cancer. In addition to the studies that have been done from within a reductionistic framework (ones in which answers are sought by breaking substances down into their smallest particles), there also is an understanding in TCM that fatty foods create heat in the system, which exceeds humans' needs given their ecological situation. Eskimos eat large amounts of fat because their bodies need to produce high amounts of heat. When average Americans eat the same amount of fat as Eskimos, they most likely will develop severe cholesterol problems. Furthermore, too much heat in the system creates an imbalance between hot and cold, or *Yin* and *Yang*, according to TCM. When this balance is disrupted, problems in the bioenergy system begin to manifest.

Sugars

Like saturated fats, refined sugars cause imbalances in the body when eaten in excess. Refined sugars are the simple sugars such as white, raw, brown, or turbinado sugar, as well as honey, corn syrup, corn sweeteners, dextrose, and fructose. Although a sweet flavor has a strengthening effect on the digestive system, according to TCM, it must come from complex carbohydrates, such as grains, fruits, and beans. Unlike the refined carbohydrates, these foods provide a more lasting energy, facilitating a more balanced physical, emotional, and intellectual experience every day. Foods filled with refined sugars create an excess in the system, as they overstimulate the endocrine system in the production of enzymes and hormones to deal with the sudden onslaught of glucose into the cells. When cookies, cakes, candies, ice cream, and other foods laden with refined sugars are consumed, an initial burst of energy occurs and shortly thereafter a feeling of fatigue and lethargy. This kind of eating pattern, when continued for a period of time, can negatively affect health because it stresses the endocrine system unnecessarily.

KEY POINT

Fresh fruit and malt barley, rice syrup, or blackstrap molasses are good to use as sweeteners because as complex sugars they stress the body less.

Dairy

Dairy is another important group to consider. Although milk is touted as the complete food by the dairy industry, it is not without its problems. Dairy products can negatively affect the mucous membranes and contribute to digestive difficulties. Humankind is the only species that drinks milk as adults and milk of a different species no less. According to TCM, excess consumption of dairy produces a condition called *dampness*, displayed as abdominal distention, edema, cysts, and allergies.

Energetic Quality of Food

A quality of food that often is overlooked during the assessment of nutritional needs is that of energy. Considering that the human organism is an aggregate of physical and chemical components that has been given form by an energy system, it can be understood that the living substance of food also has energetic properties. For example, the energetic quality of a hot red pepper is obviously different from that of a green cucumber, the former being hot and producing a diaphoretic effect (inducing perspiration) on the system, whereas the latter is wet and cool and producing a diuretic (need to urinate) effect. The more people note cravings of particular foods and the effects of foods on their bodies, the more they will become aware of the subtle qualities of foods and how these foods affect digestion and general level of energy. The ultimate aim is to eat only those foods that facilitate good health, which will vary at different times. For instance, in the winter, when they are suffering cold symptoms, it is useful for people to consume hot or warming foods, such as foods spiced with ginger and cayenne pepper, whereas in the middle of a hot, sticky summer, the consumption of cold foods, such as lettuce, cucumbers, and fruits such as watermelon is preferable.

A Healthy Diet

Recognizing that each individual is unique, some general recommendations can be followed to promote health and well-being. First, it is important to consider the times of day that food is eaten. It is generally not a good idea to skip breakfast, as it provides the foundation for the day. Eating a hot breakfast such as oatmeal or any other warm cereal or toast in the morning creates a warming and nourishing effect and supplies necessary energy to sustain daily activities. It is best to eat the heaviest meal in the middle of the day when the digestive energies are the strongest. Eating while in a rush or while conducting business is not a good practice; taking the time to eat in a relaxed manner without being engaged in any other activity is more healthful. In general, fresh organic foods (foods not treated with pesticides, hormones, and antibiotics) are good choices. A basic food guide is provided in Table 1-2. Natural vitamins and food supplements can provide additional benefits (see Chapter 3 on nutritional supplements for more information about this).

Exercise

Reviewing the type and frequency of exercise is a significant component of the assessment of health habits. It is important to evaluate whether the right kind of exercise for the body is being done on a regular basis.

The proper quantity and quality of exercise are essential for good health. Exercise needs to be part of the daily routine to offer maximum benefit. A good exercise program is one

---

TABLE 1-2 Basic Daily Food Plan

Breakfast
- Warm cereals, whole-grain muffin, or toast
- Fresh fruit
- Herbal tea or a grain beverage such as Postum, Cafix, or Bambu (1 cup of coffee a day)

Lunch
- Fresh organic salads
- Homemade soup or a sandwich made with organic turkey, chicken, hard-boiled organic eggs, or nut butter on whole-grain bread
- Fresh fruit

Dinner
- Protein, such as organic poultry, fish, beef (not more than once a month), or beans
- A complex carbohydrate, such as a vegetable, whole grains, peas, and beans
- Organic vegetables (meaning they are free of contaminants, synthetic pesticides and herbicides, hormones, preservatives, and artificial coloring)
- Fresh fruit

that is well rounded and contains components that will develop the body's musculature, improve and increase metabolic rate, and establish a balanced, uninterrupted flow of energy. A combination of aerobic exercise, weight training, and energy-based exercises, such as Hatha Yoga and T'ai Chi Kung, are a good plan. (For more information on exercise, see Chapter 4: Exercise: Mindfulness in Movement.)

KEY POINT

A lack of exercise results in weakness and atrophy of muscles, skeletal misalignment, reduced circulation of blood and energy, and poor metabolism.

Elimination

The body must eliminate waste products to maintain health. Urinary and bowel elimination should regularly occur without strain or discomfort. Normally, bowel movements should occur without the use of laxatives or enemas. If constipation is a recurring problem, it would be important to examine diet, activity, and time allocated for bowel elimination. Chronic constipation or diarrhea indicates a problem that warrants evaluation.

Rest and Sleep

People need to retreat from activity and stimulation to refresh and renew their reserves. Although variation can exist among individuals, on the daily average, adults need about eight hours of sleep. A short daytime nap also can be helpful in refreshing the body. Rather than basing the assessment of rest and sleep just on the hours sleeping, people need to look for signs that their sleep requirements are not being met. These could include the following:

- Difficulty awakening in the morning or feeling groggy on awakening rather than refreshed
- Frequent yawning
- Sleepiness throughout the day and a tendency to "nod off" when sitting inactively for awhile
- Fatigue

If signs of a sleep problem are identified, factors contributing to it need to be explored. Such factors would include the following:

- Time allocated for sleep
- Activity level throughout the day
- Caffeine and alcohol consumption

- Eating pattern before bedtime
- Stress-producing activities before bedtime
- Snoring and other disruptions from person sharing one's bed
- Environmental factors (light, noise, and room temperature)

Plans to correct sleep problems will be based on the identified factors.

Stress Patterns and Coping Mechanisms

Stress, a phenomenon associated with tension and a sense of urgency, is experienced by more and more people every day in response to an extremely complex social and economic world. Even children are not exempt from this experience, as evidenced by the increasing numbers of children with attention deficit disorder, attention deficit hyperactive disorder, asthma, and other stress-related conditions.

To gain some insight into their stress level, people should be advised to take a few minutes to self-evaluate, using a tool such as that shown in Table 1-3. As these questions

---

TABLE 1-3 Taking Stock of Your Stress Patterns

- How do you talk? Do you tend to talk fast and/or loud?
- How do you make decisions? Do you make them in a slow and deliberate way, or quickly to get them done with?
- Do you let people finish what they are saying before you speak (especially people close to you, such as family and friends)?
- Do you consider sitting alone quietly to think or practice a relaxation or meditation exercise a waste of time?
- Do you feel that you have enough time to finish your work when expected?
- Do you multitask?
- Do you tend to feel impatient when doing routine tasks, such as writing checks, filling out forms, or washing dishes?
- Do you skip meals or shortchange sleep to have more time to get things done?
- Do you feel satisfied with your current position and status at your job?
- Do you feel satisfied with your relationships?
- Do you become irritable when waiting in line or stuck in traffic?
- Do you enjoy a challenging competition?
- Do you react to most problems in an easy-going manner?
- Do you experience symptoms (e.g., palpitations, headache, insomnia) when stressed?

are answered, people should be encouraged to reflect on their answers to gain insight into their level of tension and its effect on overall health and well-being. It is essential to understand the motivation behind behaviors in order to be able to change. For instance, does a person speak loudly because he or she feels angry and requires that people give their full attention or because he or she is anxious and the tension in the chest and throat is such that it manifests as a loud and forceful voice? After the behavior is recognized, its causes can be explored. The more information that people have about their behavior and its underlying motivations, the more ammunition they have for change and attaining optimum health.

The person who becomes irritable while standing in a slow line or being stuck in traffic may be seeing only the negative aspects of waiting. Waiting provides a wonderful opportunity to practice relaxation techniques such as being present in the moment, which is a concept found in ancient Eastern teachings. To be present in the moment, one has to put aside worries and anxieties for the sake of the experience of a calmer state. The level of stress is directly proportional to the way one perceives the world. If it is perceived that there is not enough time, a person will feel harried, whereas when there is the belief that there is ample time to accomplish a task, one is relaxed. Table 1-4 offers some pointers for acquiring relaxation skills.

TABLE 1-4   Learning to Relax

In addition to becoming aware of attitudes that color your perceptions, you also can benefit by developing relaxation skills. There are four areas involved with acquiring relaxation skills:

1. *Place and time of practice.* Relaxation exercises are best done in a quiet environment at the same time each day. This helps to make the exercise part of the daily routine.

2. *Posture.* The idea is that your body becomes as relaxed as possible without falling asleep. When you sit, it is important that the head and neck are aligned with the rest of the spine to ensure the proper flow of energy.

3. *Cultivation of the right attitude.* Having the proper attitude is very important. When you first make an intentional effort to relax you may feel anxious and you need to try to put aside your worries and anxiety conscientiously while you practice the relaxation technique. It is understandable that an untrained mind will wander, but as you return your attention to the exercise you are engaged in, you will gain control over your mind more and more.

4. *Directing attention.* The practice of relaxation is impossible without directing your attention. This means that as you make the effort to concentrate and return your wandering mind to the object of concentration you are developing the ability to focus on any object or activity or idea without being sidetracked by passing thoughts or external events.

Summary

Self-care refers to the active role individuals assume in maintaining and improving their health. In Western medicine, self-care primarily implies preventing illness and recognizing symptoms early; however, TCM views health in terms of sufficient free-flowing energy circulating freely within a person. An ideal health profile is one in which a person consumes an appropriate quality and quantity of food, exercises regularly, maintains weight within an ideal range, has good stress coping skills, balances work and play, looks forward to activities with energy and enthusiasm, falls asleep easily and sleeps well, eliminates waste with ease, enjoys a satisfying sex life, feels a sense of purpose, and is free of pain and other symptoms.

REFLECTION

In taking stock of your overall personal health habits, what specific actions can you take to improve your health?

Assessment entails more than identifying abnormalities. Factors impacting health state also must be explored, which include eating patterns, factors related to eating, and quality and quantity of food intake, type and frequency of exercise, decision-making, speech pattern, ability to relax, satisfaction with work and relationships, and reactions to circumstances. People need to understand underlying factors affecting their health state so that they can develop individualized plans that address their unique situations.

Suggested Reading

Bravata, D. M., Smith-Spangler, C., Sundaram, V., Gienger, A. L., Lin, N., Lewis, R., et al. (2007). Using pedometers to increase physical activity and improve health: a systematic review. *Journal of the American Medical Association, 298*(19):2296–2304.

Callaghan, D. M. (2003). Health-promoting self-care behaviors, self-care self-efficacy, and self-care. *Nursing Science Quarterly, 16*(3):247–254.

Clark, C. C. (2003). *American Holistic Nurses' Association Guide to Common Chronic Conditions. Self-Care Options to Complement Your Doctor's Advice.* Hoboken, NJ: John Wiley and Sons.

Forkner-Dunn, J. (2003). Internet-based patient self-care: The next generation of health care delivery. *Journal of Medical Internet Research, 5*(2):e8.

Funnell, M. M., & Anderson, R.M. (2003). Patient empowerment: A look back, a look ahead. *Diabetes Education, 29*(3):454–458, 460, 462.

Halcon, L. L., Robertson, C. L., Monson, K. A., & Claypatch, C. C. (2007). A theoretical framework for using health realization to reduce stress and improve coping in refugee communities. *Journal of Holistic Nursing, 25*(3):186–194.

Hertz, J. E., & Anschutz, C. A. (2002). Relationships among perceived enactment of autonomy, self-care, and holistic health in community-dwelling older adults. *Journal of Holistic Nursing, 20*(2):166–185.

Kim, H. (2007). *Handbook of Oriental Medicine*, 3rd ed. San Francisco: Harmony and Balance Press.

Lu, H. C. (2006). *Traditional Chinese Medicine*. Laguna Beach, CA: Basic Health Publications.

Murray, R. B., & Zentner, J. P. (2000). *Health Promotion Strategies Through the Lifespan*, 7th ed. New York: Prentice Hall.

Oyserman, D., Fryberg, S. A., & Yoder, N. (2007). Identity-based motivation and health. *Journal of Personality and Social Psychology*, *93*(6):1011–1027.

Son, J. S., Kerstetter, D. L., Yarnal, C., & Baker, B. L. (2007). Promoting older women's health and well-being through social leisure environments: what we have learned from the Red Hat Society. *Journal of Women and Aging*, *19*(3–4):89–104.

Spero, D. (2002). *The Art of Getting Well: A Five Step Plan for Maximizing Health When You Have a Chronic Illness*. Alameda, CA: Hunter House.

Sutherland, J. A. (2000). Getting to the point. *American Journal of Nursing*, *100*(9):40–45.

Chapter 2

Healthful Nutrition

OBJECTIVES

This chapter should enable you to

· Define nutrition
· Discuss factors related to the emotional, psychological, cultural, and traditional aspects of food
· Outline a sample, 1-month plan to change eating habits
· List the components of a food journal
· Describe a healthy style for meal intake
· Outline recommended dietary intake according to the Food Guide Pyramid
· Give at least two examples of equivalent servings from the bread, vegetable, fruit, dairy, meat, and fat groups
· Describe the information that can be found on Nutrition Facts labels
· Define macronutrients and micronutrients
· List at least six tips for good nutrition

Sensible nutrition is a primary factor in leading a life that will allow for ample energy, productivity, and overall health. The old common sense adage "you are what you eat" is now regarded as definitive, scientific-based knowledge. In fact, the last decade has seen an explosion of data, information, and scientific research in the areas of nutrition and nutritional supplementation. The results continue to demonstrate that the foods we eat determine health, well-being, and longevity and that some foods offer medicinal qualities—something our foremothers and forefathers knew hundreds, even thousands of years ago!

Consumers are increasingly aware of the importance of nutrition to their health and are working to improve this area of their lives; nevertheless, many people believe eating nutriously will mean sacrifices, such as having to invest more time and money and forfeit good taste in order to eat healthfully. The overload of nutrition information from the media is leading many people to simply give up thinking about their nutrition and diet altogether. Moreover, food companies run 60-second commercials that promote 60-second meals. The focus keeps us eating certain foods for their taste, texture, and quick preparation time rather than their nutritive value. Americans have lowered their fat and salt intakes yet continue to have a considerable gap between recommended dietary patterns and what they actually eat.

KEY POINT

The idea that balanced nutrition is directly related to health, wellness, longevity, and the ability to heal the body is ageless. During the Stone Age, plants were used for medicinal purposes; the Chinese have used food for prevention and cures for centuries. Hippocrates was at the forefront of holistic health and wellness by suggesting that diet and nature should be taken into account when treating illness. Florence Nightingale also believed that "selecting and preparing healing foods, in addition to fresh air, quiet, and 'punctuality and care in administration of diet'" were necessary to keep the body working properly and for healing in times of injury or illness.[1] Samuel Hahnemann,[2] the father of homeopathy, believed that including foods that were most medicinal was integral to health and wellness. These great minds had an innate understanding that nutrition was directly related to health, wellness, and healing.

What Is Nutrition?

Nutrition refers to the ingestion of foods and the relationship of food to human health. Sensible nutrition requires the intake of nutrients from good quality, wholesome foods that support and maintain health throughout the lifespan. The need for sensible nutrition is essential throughout life because all humans require the same basic nutrients no matter what their stage of life. What varies is the amount of nutrients needed at each growth stage. There are also special needs because of growth and development, pregnancy and lactation, age, and disease or injury.

Proper nutrition works primarily through sound food choices. In order for proper digestion, absorption, metabolism, and elimination to take place, you must have high-quality food that contains optimum nutrients.

KEY POINT

Nutrients are substances the body needs to provide you with energy, allow you to maintain your health, and repair and regenerate your tissues and cells.

Nutrients are not immediately available as your food as eaten but must be broken down by the digestive process and taken by the blood and lymph to be used as needed, and finally, their waste must be eliminated. The food you put on your plate must be worked into proper condition and shape for use by the body. In other words, it must be digested. This begins the process; then it must be further assimilated, metabolized, and finally eliminated.

Eating slowly and with few distractions, masticating (chewing) the food thoroughly, and drinking (any beverage) minimally during meals, will allow the gastric juices to accomplish their proper function, and healthy digestion can occur. If food is swallowed nearly whole, a longer time will be required for its digestion and assimilation.

KEY POINT

Imagine the body as a group of workmen who are building a house. Each substance (food), like pieces of wood, must be cut to just the right size (chewing) and prepared for use (digestion). Next, these pieces (nutrients), after due preparation in the workshop, must be taken by the different groups of workmen (blood and lymph) to its appropriate locality in the house (muscles, organs, tissues, and cells), and there it is fitted into its proper place—this is assimilation.

Refuel, Reload, Rejuvenate

Energy is the most important reason to keep the body nutritionally sound. Each day you must refuel the body so that it can move and work. The body is continually undergoing changes; worn-out tissues and cells are constantly being repaired and renewed. The elimination of digestive waste continually requires new supplies of energy, vitamins, minerals, and other nutrients that are derived from food. Other reasons for proper diet and nutrition include fighting infection, balancing hormones, assisting in better quality sleep, and keeping the body running smoothly in times of stress. Sensible and proper nutrition is important in fulfilling these demands.

Paramount to the value of nutrition in your life is the emotional, psychological, spiritual, cultural, and traditional aspects of food. How food is presented, its smell, taste, and the emotional climate as a meal is eaten all have a connection to how food is digested. Many people use food to help ward off anxiety, tension, depression, or boredom. Certain negative feelings can cause a physiological (bodily) response in which the hypothalamus (the brain's appetite control center) sets up a chain reaction in the autonomic (self-controlling) nervous system. Additionally, the meaning food has for each individual, from early childhood experiences to the present, and how that impacts nutritional and digestive habits must also be considered.

REFLECTION

How do your food preferences and eating patterns relate to your childhood experiences?

All of the senses are stimulated when you eat through the

- Visual presentation of the food
- Surroundings in which the food is consumed
- Aroma or odor associated with the food
- Texture and taste of the food
- Conversation and environmental sounds that are present while the food is being consumed

The chemical reactions that take place in the body differ according to the combination of experiences. A delicious meal with friends that is filled with beautiful sights and sounds will elicit calmness and ease of the digestive process. Relaxing, enjoyable meals are a goal to work toward for health and wellness.

Consistency in your life, whether positive or negative, usually reigns. If food is consistently eaten quickly, poorly, and under stressful conditions, then the body, mind, and spirit will be quickly depleted, lack energy, and eventually become stressed, unhappy, uncomfortable, and diseased.

The gathering, preparing, eating, and sharing of food offer more than just nutritional value. Food and diet have social and cultural aspects. Traditions, family gatherings, and religious ceremonies that include food probably have been part of your life on a regular basis. These activities help you to carry on tradition, culture, and values. Food is considered an expression of your individuality, history, values, and beliefs. Nutrition then is much more than what food group is eaten on any particular day at any particular meal.

KEY POINT

From June Cleaver to Micky D's
As late as the 1950s many people were consuming food that was grown locally, bought fresh, and eaten in a mindful, respectful, and unstressed atmosphere. Today, you may find yourself eating in your car, on a bench at a sporting event, standing at the kitchen counter or refrigerator, or as you are walking from one meeting to the next. The demand for convenience in eating has skyrocketed to the point that more than 40% of our food expenditure is for food outside the home.[3]

Small Changes Can Make Big Differences

The adage "it's never too late" applies well to changing nutrition habits. A few small changes, in increments, can make a huge difference. The goal is to develop a pattern of healthier eating, using varied foods, in a relaxed manner. A person can begin with two to three new actions that are easy to implement and repeat them over a week or so. By the following week, another two to three new, small actions can be added to the first week's changes. This helps make these small changes easy to adapt and a routine part of everyday eating. A person can make a basic 1-month plan that incorporates these ideas:

Week 1. Cut down on portion size and begin paying attention to what you are eating.

Week 2. Eat less fat—switch to skim milk if you drink 1% or to 1% if you drink 2%. Use reduced fat or nonfat salad dressings. Cut back on cheese using 1-ounce amounts on sandwiches, or use lower fat and fat-free cheeses (1% cottage cheese, nonfat hard cheese, or part-skim mozzarella).

Week 3. Add more vegetables in an array of colors. Use the salad bar at your local supermarket if time is a factor. Eat one or two more fruits from a different color group than usual. Keep a small fruit bowl with small packs of applesauce, raisins, or other dried fruit on the kitchen counter, table, or on your desk in the office.

Week 4. Plan what small changes you will make for next month. If you followed all of the steps for these four weeks, then continue by using the Nutritional Lifestyle Survey (see Table 1-1). If you did not incorporate all the ideas for this month, then implement those that you missed this week.

A Nutritional Evaluation

Keeping a food journal for a week or two is a great help. It can be simple—consisting of a small pocket-sized notebook in which items can be jotted down such as

- What is eaten
- When it is eaten
- Where it is eaten
- Who is present when the food is eaten
- What feelings are experienced related to the food and eating experience

A food journal can be of great assistance in finding established patterns that are occurring (see Chapter 1 on assessing health habits for more discussion of nutritional assessment).

The Tune-Up

Good general health requires that there be balance in all areas of life—mind, body, spirit, family, and community. Physically it means that you eat healthful foods that provide energy and balance, without the problems of overeating, indigestion, or food intolerances. Psychologically and spiritually it means that you enjoy meals in peace, cherish and respect your food and those you share it with, and practice intention (belief and faith that all is right and

TABLE 2-1 Vitamins

Vitamin	Deficiency may cause	How it works
A	Night blindness, skin problems, dry, inflamed eyes	bone and teeth growth, vision, keeps cells, skin and tissues working properly
B-1 Thiamin	Tiredness, weakness, loss of appetite, emotional upset, nerve damage to legs (late sign)	Helps release food nutrients and energy, appetite control, helps nervous system, and digestive tract
B-2 Riboflavin	Cracks at corners of mouth, sensitivity to light, eye problems, inflamed mouth	Helps enzymes in releasing energy from cells, promotes growth, cell oxidation
Niacin	General fatigue, digestive disorders, irritability, loss of appetite, skin disorders	Fat, carbohydrate and protein metabolism, good skin, tongue and digestive system, circulation
B-6 Pyridoxine	Dermatitis, weakness, convulsions in infants, insomnia, poor immune response, sore tongue, confusion, irritability	Necessary protein metabolism, nervous system functions, formation of red blood cells, immune system function
Biotin	Rarely seen since it can be made in body if not consumed. Flaky skin, loss of appetite, nausea.	Cofactor with enzymes for metabolism of macronutrients, formation of fatty acids, helps other B vitamins be utilized
Folic Acid	Anemia, diarrhea, digestive upset, bleeding gums,	red blood cell formation, healthy pregnancy, metabolism of proteins
B12 Cobalamin	Elderly, vegetarians, or those with malabsorption disorder are at risk of deficiency-pernicious anemia, nerve damage	Necessary to form blood cells, proper nerve function, metabolism of carbohydrates and fats, builds genetic material
Pantothenic Acid	Not usually seen; vomiting, cramps, diarrhea, fatigue, tingling hands and feet, difficult coordination	Needed for many processes in the body, converts nutrients into energy, formation of some fats, vitamin utilization, making hormones

Excess may cause	Best foods to eat
Birth defects, bone fragility, vision and liver problems	Eggs, dark green and deep orange fruits and vegetables, liver, whole milk
Headache, rapid pulse, irritability, trembling, insomnia, interference with B2, B6	Whole grains and enriched breads, cereals, dried beans, pork, most vegetables, nuts, peas
No known toxic effect Some antibiotics can interfere with B2 being absorbed	whole grains, enriched bread and cereals, leafy green vegetables, diary, eggs, yogurt
Flushing, stomach pain, nausea, eye damage, can lead to heart and liver damage	Whole wheat, poultry, milk, cheese, nuts, potatoes, tuna, eggs
Reversible nerve injury, difficulty walking, numbness, impaired senses	Wheat and rice bran, fish, lean meats, whole grains, sunflower seeds, corn, spinach, bananas
Symptoms similar to vitamin B1 overdose	Egg yolks, organ meats, vegetables, fish, nuts, seeds, also made in intestines by normal bacteria there
Excessive intake can mask B12 deficiency and interfere with zinc absorption	Green leafy vegetables, organ meats, dried beans
None known except those born with defect to absorb	Liver, salmon, fish, lean meats, milk, all animal products
Rare	Lean meats, whole grains, legumes

(continues)

TABLE 2-1 **Vitamins** *(continued)*

Vitamin	Deficiency may cause	How it works
C Ascorbic Acid	Bleeding gums, slow healing, poor immune response, aching joints, nose bleeds, anemia	Helps heal wounds, collagen maintenance, resistance to infection, formation of brain chemicals
D	Poor bone growth, rickets, osteoporosis, bone softening, muscle twitches	Calcium and phosphorus, metabolism and absorption, bone and teeth formation
E	Not usually seen, after prolonged impairment of fat absorption, neurological abnormalities	Maintains cell membranes, assists as antioxidant, red blood cell formation
K	Tendency to hemorrhage, liver damage	Needed for prothrombin, blood clotting, works with Vitamin D in bone growth

as it should be) to a higher power. Family and community are areas where traditions and events usually occur with food and eating. Family get-togethers and social events are ways for us to feel connected to others; however, if established patterns of eating are not beneficial to general health, some changes may be necessary.

A Nutritional Lifestyle for the Ages

The holistic approach to nutrition and diet considers self-care, healthful food selection, moderate intake, and balance. It suggests listening to one's own inner wisdom, being present (paying attention to what is happening at the present), and following a healthful lifestyle and a diet that includes foods that work in synergy (together) with other aspects of life.

Nutritional Intake

A varied, balanced diet from wholesome, quality foods will provide much of what is needed to live a healthy, productive, long life. Varying colors, tastes, textures, and temperatures from good quality, organic food will yield the best results.

Time should be taken at meals to enjoy food, masticate (chew) it, and allow the action of the digestive powers to be fully utilized. Relaxation, enjoyable company, tranquility of mind, and pleasant conversation while eating help to fulfill the psychological, social, and

Excess may cause	Best foods to eat
Diarrhea, kidney stones, blood problems, urinary problems	Most fruits, especially citrus fruits, melon, berries, and vegetables
Headache, fragile bones, high blood pressure, increased cholesterol, calcium deposits	Egg yolks, organ meats, fortified milk, also made in skin when exposed to sun
	Vegetable oils and margarine, wheat germ, nuts, dark green vegetables, whole grains
Jaundice (yellow skin) with synthetic form, flushing & sweating	Green vegetables, oats, rye, dairy

cultural needs associated with food intake. The spiritual aspects of eating can be addressed through rituals and family traditions that are incorporated into each day's meals.

REFLECTION

Do you have rituals—such as prayer, candle lighting, or sharing time—that you incorporate into your main meals with significant others in your life? If not, how could you incorporate at least one?

Regular Meals

Consistency of food intake is important. The body must have intervals of rest from eating or its energies are soon exhausted, resulting in impaired function, dyspepsia (stomach upset), and other problems. Constant munching, whether on pastries and candy or apples and carrots, will lead to a digestive tract that is almost constantly at work; poor and weak digestion will follow, causing nutritional imbalances. Six small meals, beginning with a good breakfast is best. Meals should be approached with an attitude of self-caring that will allow the mind, body, and spirit a much needed respite from the regular schedule.

EXHIBIT 2-1   **Smart Snacking**

Instead of	Try
Potato chips or pretzels	Mini bagels or breadsticks
A candy bar	A piece of fruit or a glass of juice
Cookies	Graham crackers or raisins
Fried meats	Baked or grilled meats
Whole milk	Skim or 1% or 2% milk
Butter or syrup on pancakes	Fresh fruit
Ice cream	Frozen low-fat or light yogurt
French fries or home fries	Baked potato with herbs
Sour cream on baked potato	Nonfat yogurt and chives
Butter or cheese on vegetables	Lemon juice or herbs

Amount and Timing

People generally eat too much rather than too little. It is an excellent plan to rise from the table before the desire for food is quite satisfied. The body's nutrition does not depend on the amount eaten but on the *quality* of food consumed (see Exhibit 2-1). Eating too much is nearly as bad as swallowing food before it is properly chewed. Those who dine late should wait two or three hours before retiring. Late-evening meals usually lead to a poor night's rest, with organs such as the liver being unable to detoxify properly.

The Food Guide Pyramid and Other Helpers

The Food Guide Pyramid (see Figure 2-1), the Nutrition Facts label (see Figure 2-2), and Dietary Guidelines (see Figure 2-3) are set forth by the Food and Nutrition Board of the National Academies of Science and serve as tools to put sensible nutrition and diet choices into practice. These guidelines offer a way to eat less fat and consume a diet high in plant foods and low in animal foods. Becoming familiar with the Food Guide Pyramid, looking at the labels of the food you buy, and understanding the Dietary Guidelines are simple yet empowering. The key is to choose the foods from each group that will provide an individualized, tasty, nutrient balance and at the same time fit your lifestyle, food preferences, and cultural needs.

The Food Guide Pyramid translates the recommended dietary allowances (RDAs) and Dietary Guidelines for Americans into the kinds and number of servings of food to eat each day. The Food Guide Pyramid can be used to help you make food choices from the five

Figure 2-1   MyPyramid

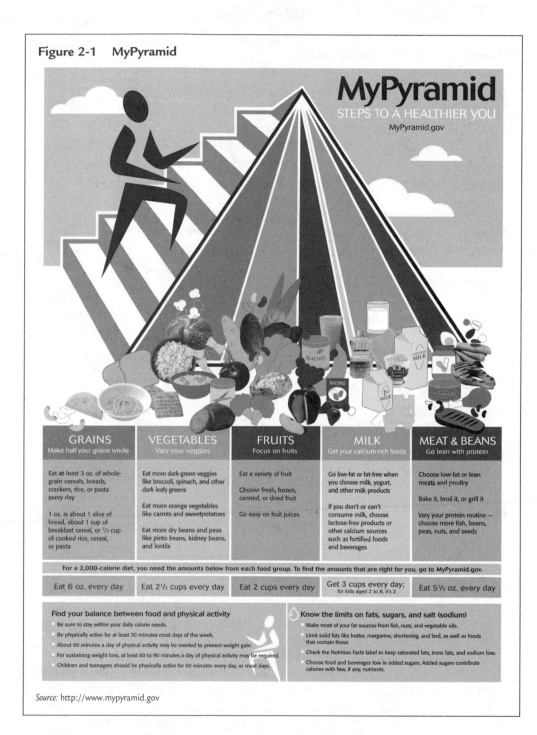

Source: http://www.mypyramid.gov

Figure 2-2 The Nutrition Facts Label

Ingredients: Wheat flour, sugar, rolled oats, corn sweetener, molasses, partially hydrogenated safflower oil, salt, pantothenic acid, reduced iron, yellow No. 6, yellow No. 5, pyridoxine, ascorbic acid (vitamin C), BHT, riboflavin, folic acid.

Figure 2-3 2005 Dietary Guidelines for Americans: Key Recommendations for the General Population

Adequate Nutrients Within Calorie Needs

· Consume a variety of nutrient-dense foods and beverages within and among the basic food groups while choosing foods that limit the intake of saturated and trans-fats, cholesterol, added sugars, salt, and alcohol.

· Meet recommended intakes within energy needs by adopting a balanced eating pattern, such as the U.S. Department of Agriculture (USDA) Food Guide or the Dietary Approaches to Stop Hypertension (DASH) Eating Plan.

Weight Management

· To maintain body weight in a healthy range, balance calories from foods and beverages with calories expended.

· To prevent gradual weight gain over time, make small decreases in food and beverage calories and increase physical activity.

Physical Activity

· Engage in regular physical activity and reduce sedentary activities to promote health, psychological well-being, and a healthy body weight.

· To reduce the risk of chronic disease in adulthood: Engage in at least 30 minutes of moderate-intensity physical activity, above usual activity, at work or home on most days of the week.

· For most people, greater health benefits can be obtained by engaging in physical activity of more vigorous intensity or longer duration.

· To help manage body weight and prevent gradual, unhealthy body weight gain in adulthood: Engage in approximately 60 minutes of moderate- to vigorous-intensity activity on most days of the week while not exceeding caloric intake requirements.

(continues)

Figure 2-3   2005 Dietary Guidelines for Americans: Key Recommendations for the General Population *(continued)*

· To sustain weight loss in adulthood: Participate in at least 60 to 90 minutes of daily moderate-intensity physical activity while not exceeding caloric intake requirements. Some people may need to consult with a healthcare provider before participating in this level of activity.

· Achieve physical fitness by including cardiovascular conditioning, stretching exercises for flexibility, and resistance exercises or calisthenics for muscle strength and endurance.

Food Groups to Encourage

· Consume a sufficient amount of fruits and vegetables while staying within energy needs. Two cups of fruit and 2 1/2 cups of vegetables per day are recommended for a reference 2000-calorie intake, with higher or lower amounts depending on the calorie level.

· Choose a variety of fruits and vegetables each day. In particular, select from all five vegetable subgroups (dark green, orange, legumes, starchy vegetables, and other vegetables) several times a week.

· Consume 3 or more ounce-equivalents of whole-grain products per day, with the rest of the recommended grains coming from enriched or whole-grain products. In general, at least half the grains should come from whole grains.

· Consume 3 cups per day of fat-free or low-fat milk or equivalent milk products.

Fats

· Consume less than 10% of calories from saturated fatty acids and less than 300 mg/day of cholesterol, and keep trans-fatty acid consumption as low as possible.

· Keep total fat intake between 20–35% of calories, with most fats coming from sources of polyunsaturated and monounsaturated fatty acids, such as fish, nuts, and vegetable oils.

· When selecting and preparing meat, poultry, dry beans, and milk or milk products, make choices that are lean, low-fat, or fat-free.

· Limit intake of fats and oils high in saturated and/or trans-fatty acids, and choose products low in such fats and oils.

Carbohydrates

· Choose fiber-rich fruits, vegetables, and whole grains often.

· Choose and prepare foods and beverages with little added sugars or caloric sweeteners, such as amounts suggested by the USDA Food Guide and the DASH Eating Plan.

· Reduce the incidence of dental caries by practicing good oral hygiene and consuming sugar- and starch-containing foods and beverages less frequently.

(continues)

Figure 2-3   2005 Dietary Guidelines for Americans: Key Recommendations for the General Population *(continued)*

Sodium and Potassium

· Consume less than 2300 mg (approximately one teaspoon of salt) of sodium per day.

· Choose and prepare foods with little salt. At the same time, consume potassium-rich foods, such as fruits and vegetables.

Alcoholic Beverages

· Those who choose to drink alcoholic beverages should do so sensibly and in moderation—defined as the consumption of up to one drink per day for women and up to two drinks per day for men.

· Alcoholic beverages should not be consumed by some individuals, including those who cannot restrict their alcohol intake, women of childbearing age who may become pregnant, pregnant and lactating women, children and adolescents, individuals taking medications that can interact with alcohol, and those with specific medical conditions.

· Alcoholic beverages should be avoided by individuals engaging in activities that require attention, skill, or coordination, such as driving or operating machinery.

Food Safety to avoid microbial foodborne illness:

· Clean hands, food contact surfaces, and fruits and vegetables. Meat and poultry should not be washed or rinsed.

· Separate raw, cooked, and ready-to-eat foods while shopping, preparing, or storing foods.

· Cook foods to a safe temperature to kill microorganisms.

· Chill (refrigerate) perishable food promptly and defrost foods properly.

· Avoid raw (unpasteurized) milk or any products made from unpasteurized milk, raw or partially cooked eggs or foods containing raw eggs, raw or undercooked meat and poultry, unpasteurized juices, and raw sprouts.

Note: The Dietary Guidelines for Americans 2005 contains additional recommendations for specific populations.

Source: From the U.S. Department of Agriculture, 2005. Available: http://www.healthierus.gov/dietaryguidelines

---

food groups. It is an excellent way to begin looking at your eating and nutrition habits and can be a starting point to making necessary changes in diet and eating for a healthier life. With the help of the pyramid you can meet your nutrient needs while selecting foods that satisfy your taste preferences. Balance, variety, and moderation are the key to these guidelines.

The shape of the pyramid illustrates the importance of balance and variety among the food groups. It is a visual presentation of the daily servings of food that should be selected with the amount of servings to be taken from each group.

Beginning at the base of the pyramid there is the *bread* group, which are the foods that form the foundation of the diet. This group includes bread, cereals, rice, and pasta. There should be 6 to 11 servings per day from this group, chosen from whole-grain products whenever possible.

One serving of bread could include:

- 1 slice of bread
- 1/2 cup of rice or pasta
- 1/2 cup cooked cereal
- 1 ounce of ready-to-eat cereal
- These should be in the form of complex carbohydrates from whole grains: wheat, oats, rye, bulgur, millet, or barley.
- Whole-grain and enriched breads, rolls, potatoes, rice, corn, and pasta.

This group also includes bagels, pancakes, biscuits, and crackers, which are not as nutrient rich as the whole grains. The poorest selections in this group are muffins, granola, fried grains or dough, and pastries. Choose foods from this group that are not refined or processed and have little or no added fats and sugars.

Next, *vegetables* that should occupy second place in amount in our daily food choices, with a minimum of three to five servings per day. Fresh vegetables are best; frozen, steamed, or baked should be the second choice. A variety of colors, from green leafy to orange, red, and yellow, should be chosen from this group.

One serving of vegetables could include:

- 3/4 cup of vegetable juice
- 1 cup raw leafy vegetables
- 1/2 cup of other vegetables, cooked or chopped raw

Fruits make up the right half of the second tier of the Food Guide Pyramid. Two to four servings per day should be consumed from this group, with fresh fruit being the primary choice and then frozen or canned in water or juice. Color and preference again should vary in this group. Grains, vegetables, and fruits comprise more than two-thirds of the pyramid, reflecting that they should make up the major portion of the daily diet.

One serving of fruit could include:

- One medium whole fresh fruit
- 1/4 cup dried fruit
- 1/2 cup chopped, cooked, or canned fruit
- 3/4 cup of fruit juice

Moving up the pyramid is the *milk* group, from which there should be two to three servings per day. Because caloric intake will depend on whether whole milk or low-fat products are used, it is best to use low-fat products unless there is a special need to consume extra calories.

One serving of milk could include:

- 1 cup of milk or yogurt
- 1 1/2 to 2 ounces of natural cheese (processed cheese is least desired)

The *meat* group includes red meats, poultry, fish, eggs, dried beans, and nuts. A hamburger bun or a deck of cards is the size of an average meat serving. Meat that is broiled or baked with all excess fat trimmed and the skin removed is best.

One serving of meat could include:

- 2 to 3 ounces of cooked lean meat, fish, or poultry
- 1/2 cup of cooked beans
- one egg
- 1/3 cup of nuts
- 2 tablespoons of peanut butter, which is equal to 1 ounce or 1/3 serving of meat

Only two servings daily from the milk and meat groups are suggested because of the high level of fats and calories that these foods tend to have. They are important to the diet for B_{12}, phosphorus, calcium, and other important nutrients, but are needed in lesser amounts than other foods.

Finally, *fats, oils, and sugars*, which are at the tip of the pyramid, should be used sparingly and only occasionally. This group provides few nutrients and is high in fat and simple sugar content. If a person is trying to lose weight or wishes to maintain his or her present weight, these foods should be limited.

Fats consumed in foods such as french fries or other fried foods count also, as do fats and oils used in cooking. Vegetable oils are preferable because they are low in saturated fat. A diet providing no more than 30% of total calories from fat is suggested: 10% from saturated fat, 10% from monounsaturated fats, and 10% from polyunsaturated fats. Because fat contains more than twice the calories of an equal serving of carbohydrates or protein, reducing fat intake will help you take in fewer calories.

Fats could include

- butter
- margarine
- cream
- cream cheese
- mayonnaise
- oils
- salad dressings
- gravy or sauces

Sugars could include

- table sugar (sucrose)
- brown sugar
- honey
- molasses
- raw sugar
- syrup

- corn sweetener
- corn syrup
- glucose
- high-fructose corn syrup
- fructose
- lactose (milk sugar)

KEY POINT

One way to calculate calories from fat is to use this simple formula:

1. Take the number of calories eaten daily
2. Multiply by 30% (the suggested percentage of calories from fat)
3. Divide the answer by 9 (the amount of calories in one gram of fat).

For example, if you eat 1500 calories per day, the equation would look like this:

$$1500 \times .30 = 450 \div 9 = 50$$

Fifty grams of unsaturated fat would be your daily intake.

The taste of sugar is appealing. Sugars are used in many processed foods, such as bakery goods, cereals, and thickeners. Sugars are also used as natural preservatives. The sugar consumed should be naturally present in fruits, grains, some vegetables, and dairy.

Exhibit 2-2 describes nutritional strategies for the Food Guide Pyramid.

Nutrition Facts Label

The regulation of food dates back to the beginning of the last century. Under regulations from the Food and Drug Administration (FDA) of the Department of Health and Human Services and the Food Safety and Inspection Service of the U.S. Department of Agriculture (USDA), the food label was designed to give more information about nutrition. By law, nearly all food labels must contain a Nutrition Facts panel that contains information as to how the food can fit into an overall daily diet.

EXHIBIT 2-2   Nutrition Strategies for the Food Guide Pyramid

·   Consume different foods from each group to improve your chances of receiving all of the nutrients that your body needs in the proper balance.

·   As you head to the checkout at the supermarket, look over your choices. If there is a Food Guide Pyramid on one of the products, use it to determine whether you have a good representation of all the foods groups in your cart: cereal, bread, rice, and pasta in good number; next a variety of types and colors of vegetables and fruit, enough for five servings per day per person; then some dairy (low fat), fish, poultry, or meat/meat alternatives; and finally, a limited number of candy, cookies, cakes, pies, or other rich desserts, chips, or salty snacks.

·   Use the Nutrition Facts label on food packages to guide you in meeting 100% of the recommended daily allowance of nutrients.

Nutrition Panel Format

The Nutrition Facts label (see Figure 2-2) on the side or back of a package states the amount of saturated fat, cholesterol, fiber, and other nutrients each serving contains. By checking the serving size on several products, you can compare the nutritional qualities of similar foods.

The "% Daily Values" on the panel is based on a 2000-calorie per day diet and shows the percentage of a nutrient provided in one portion. The aim is to meet 100% of the daily value for total carbohydrates, fiber, vitamins, and minerals listed. The percentage for fat, sodium (salt), and cholesterol can add up to less than 100. The amount of fat, cholesterol, sodium, carbohydrates, and protein (in grams or milligrams) are listed to the immediate right of these nutrients.

Nutrition at Different Life Stages

The Dietary Guidelines for Americans, the Food Guide Pyramid, and Nutrition Facts labels are meant to be used by the average adult who is healthy, active, and within the guidelines for height and weight. There are other factors that affect the amount and type of food needed daily.

Children from birth to five years require more vitamins, calcium, and other nutrients for growth and development. Dietary Guidelines generally are not meant to be used for children under two. In childhood, these guidelines can be applied, using smaller portions for younger children and increasing portions as they get older. *Adolescents, pregnant adolescents, and pregnant and lactating women* need more breads, fruit, vegetables, milk, and meat because of higher nutrient needs.

Good nutrition for those *50 years of age and older* can decrease the effects of health problems that are prevalent among older Americans. It also can improve the quality of life for people who have chronic disease. Older people are likely to have poor appetites, experience health problems, take medications, and have sedentary lifestyles. They may also limit beneficial foods because of chewing, digestive, or intestinal health problems. This may lead to poor dietary intake and nutritional imbalances.

Diversity in Nutritional Lifestyles

Ethnic cuisine is becoming more and more popular in the United States, with the Mediterranean Diet perhaps being the best-known and used alternative diet. It includes bread and pasta, vegetables, legumes, fresh fruit, breads, and some unsaturated oils (olive), a few red meats and fish, and more eggs and poultry than the U.S. Food Guide Pyramid. Garlic is usually a staple, and the food is cooked fresh with the use of other herbs for flavor. Diet pyramids have emerged for Asian, Latin American, and Vegan diets, representing what epidemiologic (development of a particular issue within a certain population) studies have associated with optimum health.

Interest in vegetarianism is increasing and leading the way for Asian, specifically Japanese, Chinese, and Native American (hunter–gatherer) diets. The Japanese diet is one of the healthiest in the world, whereas other Asian cuisines offer low-fat diets with various selections from plant and some animal (fish) foods. Some studies have suggested that these diets lower risk factors for heart disease and some cancers.

KEY POINT

Nutrients are elements of our food that make up macronutrients and micronutrients. Macronutrients are consumed in large amounts, tens and hundreds of grams (ounces and pounds). Micronutrients, minerals, and trace elements are ingested in thousandths and millionths of a gram (milligrams and micrograms). Fiber and water, although not classified as nutrients, are essential to proper nutrition, digestion, assimilation, and elimination. Although each nutrient has its own job, all nutrients work together to help the body function at optimal levels. The combined action (synergy)is far greater than if taken separately.

The Macronutrients

Macronutrients include *water, fiber, carbohydrates, protein, and fats*. These are essential for the body and mind to *work efficiently, function properly, and maintain and repair itself.*

Water

Water, not truly a macronutrient, is fundamental for life. It has a role in every major bodily function and is the substance that allows chemical reactions to occur from the nutrients we ingest. This makes it essential to proper diet and nutrition. Water maintains the body's proper temperature, transports nutrients to and toxins from the cells, lubricates our joints, transports oxygen through the blood and lymphatic systems, and comprises from one-half to two-thirds of our body. Without water, death is imminent within days. The body requires between 9 and 12 cups of pure drinking water daily, in addition to water obtained through soups, fruits, and other foods.

Tap water quality varies by locale in the United States. Various processes are used to purify water and remove major contaminants from water supplies. These processes are filtration, distillation, and reverse osmosis. The results of all water testing done by your local water supply board are part of the public record, and you can request copies of recent monitoring reports as part of the Freedom of Information Act. If you have a private well, you can have the water tested by a certified laboratory. (Refer to the resources section at the end of this chapter for information about safe water sources.)

Fiber

Like water, fiber is not a true macronutrient, although it is another important element in the nutrition equation. A diet containing a minimum of 20 to 30 grams of fiber per day is recommended. The typical American is said to eat only about 11 grams of fiber per day.

Vegetables, fruits, peas, beans, and whole grains contain fiber. Proper bowel elimination can be attained by eating fiber because it adds bulk and hastens the course of food and waste through the intestinal system. Fiber, in conjunction with a low (saturated)-fat, low-cholesterol diet, has been found to reduce the risk for heart disease, digestive disorders, certain cancers, and diabetes. The sustained absence of fiber in the diet can lead to problems of the gastrointestinal tract, including diverticular disease and constipation.

KEY POINT

Following the suggestions of the USDA's Food Guide Pyramid, eating two to four servings of fruit (fresh, unpeeled) and five servings of vegetables (some raw and unpeeled) will allow for an average of 20 to 30 grams of fiber in the diet—the recommended daily intake.

Carbohydrates

Carbohydrates provide the body with energy and are comprised of two classes: complex and simple carbohydrates. Foods that contain starches and fiber are called complex carbohydrates; sugars are simple carbohydrates. Fruits, vegetables, and grain products (breads, cereals, and pasta) are complex carbohydrates. Avoiding simple carbohydrates—foods containing added sugar such as candy, soft drinks, cookies, cakes, ice cream, and pies—will increase energy and lower risks for health problems. The body cannot differentiate between complex and simple carbohydrates; therefore, the body will metabolize candy, which has a high added sugar content (and is high in saturated fat), and a piece of fruit, which has natural sugar, the same way. The candy bar, however, contains few nutrients, and the excess sugar will be immediately stored as fat in the body. The fruit contains many required nutrients as well as fiber and will be used for energy more quickly than the candy.

Carbohydrates are necessary for protein to be digested. They provide the blood with glucose, which is formed during the digestive process and is needed by the body and brain to give energy to muscles, tissues, and organs. When carbohydrates are present in the system, the body is able to use protein for regeneration and repair.

Protein

Protein is the body's secondary energy source and has many functions. Protein must be present for the body to grow, repair damaged or injured tissue, create new tissue, and regulate water balance. It is the component that lays the foundation for major organs, blood and blood clotting, muscles, skin, hair, nails, hormones, enzymes, and antibodies. It maintains a proper balance of acid and alkaline in the blood.

KEY POINT

There are 22 amino acids, 8 of which are called "essential" amino acids and must be consumed through the diet because the body is unable to manufacture them.

The essential elements in protein are amino acids. Foods that consist of all of the essential amino acids are considered complete proteins. These usually come from meat, fish, fowl, eggs, and dairy. Those that come from vegetable sources such as beans, grain, and peas are considered incomplete proteins because they supply the body with only some of the essential amino acids.

Fats

Lipids (fats) are another source of energy for the body. The lipid group of macronutrients is vital for health but is needed in small amounts. Fats supply essential fatty acids, such as linoleic (omega-6) and linoleic acid (omega-3). They also help maintain healthy skin; regulate cholesterol metabolism; are precursors to prostaglandin (a hormone-like substance that regulates some body processes); carry fat-soluble vitamins A, D, E, and K, and aid in their absorption from the intestine; act as a cushion and stabilizer for our internal organs; and supply a protective layer that helps regulate body temperature and maintain heat. (The section on diabetes in Chapter 3 discusses essential fatty acids further.)

Fats supply greater energy than carbohydrates or protein. Fat has nine calories per gram, whereas carbohydrates and protein contain only four calories per gram. One molecule of fat can be broken down into three molecules of fatty acids and one molecule of glycerol. This structure is known chemically as triglycerides, which make up approximately 90% of all dietary fat.

Fatty acids are generally classified as saturated, monounsaturated, and polyunsaturated. In general, fats that contain a majority of saturated fatty acids are solid at room temperature. Fats containing mostly unsaturated fatty acids are usually liquid at room temperature and are called oils. *Saturated fatty acids* are found in meats, cream, whole milk, butter, cheese, coconut oil, palm kernel oil, and vegetable shortening. *Monounsaturated fatty acids* are found in olive and canola oils. *Polyunsaturated fatty acids* are found in other vegetable oils, nuts, and some fish. Both types of fatty acids, when used to replace saturated fats, can help to reduce the level of "bad" cholesterol in blood.

Cholesterol is not fat, but is rather a fat-like substance classified as a *lipid*. Cholesterol is vital to life and is found in all cell membranes. It is necessary for the production of bile acids and steroid hormones. Dietary cholesterol is found in only animal foods and is abundant in organ meats, egg yolks, meats, and poultry. Low-density lipoprotein (bad cholesterol), and high-density lipoprotein (good cholesterol), are the two types. Low-density lipoproteins are those that increase the risk of cardiovascular disease.

Because all fats contain different amounts of the three fatty acids, the ratio of polyunsaturated to saturated fats in what is eaten is important. The recommendation from the National Institutes of Health is that overall intake should be in the highest ratio of monounsaturated and polyunsaturated fats with no more than 30% of daily calories from fat sources in the diet and reducing saturated fat to less than 10% of calories.

KEY POINT

When buying foods that contain fat, be sure to read the labels. Some foods say that they are low cholesterol but are still high in fat.

The Micronutrients

Vitamins and minerals are the micronutrients (elements) in food that help the body to function properly. They are needed in trace or small amounts and occur naturally in food.

Vitamins and minerals work in synergy. This word comes from Greek *synergos*, meaning work. Synergism is the working together of all the nutrients that are in food, in the needed ratio, for the optimal functioning of the body/mind.

Vitamins and minerals should be taken in whole foods as much as possible because foods contain hundreds of compounds that assist the body to use these nutrients.

Vitamins

Vitamins do not have any calories and cannot be used as a food source, but they are necessary for life. They are needed for the body to grow, develop, maintain its metabolic processes, and assist in digestion and assimilation. Vitamins are assisted in the body by enzymes. Table 2-1 lists signs of deficiency, functions, signs of toxicity, and food sources for each vitamin.

There are two types of vitamins: water and fat soluble. Water-soluble vitamins are those that dissolve in water and are excreted through our skin (perspiration), lungs (breathing), intestines (bowel), and mainly through the kidneys (urine) if not needed or used by the body. They include the B-complex group: B_1 (thiamin), B_2 (riboflavin), B_3 (niacin), B_6 (pyridoxine), folic acid (folacin, folate, or pteroylgutamic acid {PGA}), B_{12} (cobalamin or cyanocobalamin), biotin, pantothenic acid, and vitamin C (see Table 2-1).

Each vitamin has its own function. The *B-complex* group's functions are many. They range from normal neurologic (nervous) system functioning; synthesizing (linking) nonessential amino acids; helping oxidize (burn) glucose; assisting in the digestion of carbohydrates; promoting protein metabolism; and assisting in the production of various hormones, red blood cells, and genetic materials (such as RNA and DNA).

Vitamin C (ascorbic acid) has its best known source in citrus fruits, but can also be found in most fresh fruits and vegetables, especially, tomatoes, broccoli, and potatoes. It is essential for the formation of collagen, the protein that helps form skin, bone, and ligaments. It is also needed for iron to be absorbed, to prevent hemorrhaging, to help wounds to heal, and to help with allergic reactions.

Fat-soluble vitamins attach to protein and are carried throughout the body by the blood. Unlike water-soluble vitamins, fat-soluble vitamins can be stored in the liver and adipose (fatty) tissues of the body if taken in excess. Fat-soluble vitamins include vitamins A, D, E, and K.

KEY POINT

The opportunity for toxicity is greater with fat-soluble vitamins because they are stored in the body.

Small amounts of vitamins D and K can be made by the body. The sources for these vitamins are green/deep yellow/orange vegetables, deep yellow/orange fruits, whole grains, low-fat dairy, vegetable oil, seeds, nuts, eggs, and liver. Their functions include preventing night blindness; helping vision; promoting healthy skin, hair, teeth, and nails; boosting the immune system; assisting the absorption of calcium; maintaining mucous membranes; and blood clotting.

Minerals

Minerals (Table 2-2) are further broken down into groups: *macrominerals*, those required in milligrams (larger amounts) by the body; *trace minerals*, required in micrograms (smaller

TABLE 2-2 Minerals

Minerals	Deficiency may cause	How it works
Calcium	Rickets, soft bones, osteoporosis, cramps, numbness and tingling arms and legs	Strong bones, teeth, muscle and nerve function, blood clotting
Phosphorus	Weakness and bone pain, otherwise rare	Works with calcium, helps with nerve, muscle, and heart function
Magnesium	Muscle weakness, twitching, cardiac problems, tremors, confusion, formation of blood clots,	Needed for other minerals and enzymes to work, helps bone growth, muscle contraction
Potassium	Lethargy, weakness, abnormal heart rhythm, nervous disorders	Fluid balance, controls heart, muscle, nerve, and digestive function
Iron	Anemia, weakness, fatigue, pallor, poor immune response	Forms of hemoglobin and myoglobin- supplies oxygen to cells, muscles
Iodine	Goiter, weight gain, increased risk of breast cancer	Helps metabolize fat, thyroid function
Zinc	Poor growth, poor wound healing, loss of taste, poor sexual development	Works with many enzymes for metabolism and digestion, immune support, wound healing, reproductive development
Manganese	Nerve damage, dizziness, hearing problems	Enzyme cofactor for metabolism, control blood sugar, nervous, and immune functions
Copper	Rare, but can cause anemia and growth problems in children	Enzyme activation, skin pigment, needed to form nerve and muscle fibers, red blood cells
Chromium	Impaired glucose tolerance in low blood sugar and diabetes	Glucose metabolism
Selenium	Heart muscle abnormalities, infections, digestive disturbances	Antioxidant with vitamin E, protects against cancer, helps maintain healthy heart
Molybdenium	Unknown	Element of enzymes needed for metabolism, helps store iron

Excess may cause	Best foods to eat
Confusion, lethargy, blocks iron absorption, deposits in body	Dairy, salmon and small bony fish, tofu.
Proper balance needed with calcium	Meat, poultry, fish, eggs, dairy, dried beans, whole grains
Proper balance needed with calcium, phosphorus, & vitamin D	Nuts, soybeans, dried beans, green vegetables
Vomiting, muscle weakness	Vegetables, fruits, dried beans, milk
Increased need for antioxidants, heart disorders	Red meats, fish, poultry, dried beans, eggs, leafy vegetables
Thyroid-decreased activity, enlargement	Seafood, iodized salt, kelp, lima beans
Digestive problems, fever, dizziness, anemia, kidney problems	Lean meats, fish, poultry, yogurt
High doses affect iron absorption	Nuts, whole grains, avocados
Usually by taking supplements. Liver problems, diarrhea.	Nuts, organ meats, seafood
Most Americans have low intakes	Brewer's yeast, whole grains, peanuts, clams
Nail, hair, and digestive problems, fatigue, garlic odor of breath	Meat and grains, dependent on soil in which they were raised
Gout, joint pains, copper deficiency	Beans, grains, peas, dark green vegetables

amounts) by the body; and *other trace minerals or elements*. The body is unable to synthesize minerals, and thus, they must be taken in through diet on a regular basis.

The macrominerals are calcium, magnesium, phosphorus, sodium, and potassium. The trace minerals include iron, iodine, manganese, chromium, selenium, copper, fluoride, molybdenum, boron, and zinc. These are only needed in the body in minute amounts, but if a deficiency or imbalance exists, it can lead to serious health problems and, if left unchecked, sometimes even death.

Calcium and phosphorus are the two most abundant minerals, and they work together in the body. *Calcium* is found predominately in the bones, where it is needed for structure. The bones store calcium for its release into the blood as needed. It assists in blood clotting, transmitting of nerve conduction, and helping with muscle contractions.

Phosphorus is found in nearly all cells of the body. It is used for energy production, metabolizing some vitamins and minerals, and building and renewing tissue and cells. The best source of phosphorus is animal protein, although milk and legumes also contain this mineral. Deficiencies of phosphorus are not usually seen because of its abundance in foods used by most Americans.

Magnesium is stored in bone, where it can be used by the body as needed. It is important for calcium, potassium, and vitamin D assimilation and is necessary for the relaxation phase of muscle contraction. Magnesium also assists in the proper functioning of the heart, liver, and other soft tissues.

Potassium, sodium, and chloride are the three minerals that are sometimes called electrolytes. *Potassium* is essential for life and necessary for heart, nerve, muscle, and digestive functioning. *Sodium* is necessary for the balance of fluid outside of the cells and is important in maintaining nerve and muscle conduction. Because sodium is abundant in food, there rarely is a chance of deficiency. *Chloride* mainly occurs with salt in foods and is needed by the body with sodium for fluid balance of the cells and also to digest proteins. Sodium and chloride are found together in common table salt.

The microminerals (trace elements) include iron, iodine, zinc, copper, manganese, molybdenum, selenium, fluoride, chromium, and silicon. *Iron* is a most essential mineral because it is needed to carry oxygen from the lungs to all the cells. Vitamin C helps with iron absorption from food, whereas calcium and phosphorus have been found to inhibit it. When there is too much iron in the body, it can cause liver and oxidative damage and lead to iron toxicity. Low iron levels can cause iron-deficiency anemia.

Iodine is needed in miniscule amounts in the body to maintain the thyroid gland. Deficiency is rare, but if it occurs, it leads to goiter (enlargement of the thyroid gland). Seafood and salt are high in iodine.

Every organ in the body uses zinc. *Zinc* has an effect on immune function, healing wounds, digestion, and converting vitamin A to a usable form. A zinc deficiency can lead to many problems, such as poor immune function, digestive problems, and poor growth and development. Although rare, zinc toxicity can interfere with iron absorption and alter cholesterol metabolism.

EXHIBIT 2-3   Ten Tips for Good Nutrition

1. Use the Food Guide Pyramid as a guideline for what to eat every day.

2. Read the labels on everything you consume.

3. Choose plenty of whole-grain products (bread, pasta, and cereals).

4. Eat at least five fruits and vegetables per day.

5. Choose foods low in fat, added sugars, and salt.

6. Enjoy meals (this helps them digest better).

7. Have dinner in a quiet atmosphere (eating mostly complex carbohydrates will help ease you into the evening and promote better sleep).

8. If you take dietary supplements, take them with meals.

9. Keep coffee, tea, alcohol, and carbonated beverages to a minimum.

10. Drink at least eight glasses of water per day.

Selenium has been found to work together with vitamin E as an antioxidant (see Chapter 3). Because it is found in the soil, deficiencies are rare because any plant that has been grown in selenium-rich soil provides selenium. Toxicity may occur when too much selenium is added to the diet through supplementation.

Chromium has recently been linked to insulin in controlling blood glucose levels. The American diet often is deficient in chromium, attributed to diets high in sugar and refined foods. Deficiencies in this vital mineral can lead to severe health problems.

The idea that what you eat will impact your health and longevity has been gaining momentum for decades. Scientific research seems to have finally caught up with it. The best nutritional strategy for reducing the risk of chronic disease and living a healthy productive life is to follow a basic, sensible nutritional plan, as outlined in Exhibit 2-3.

Some basic tips for good nutrition are also listed in Exhibit 2-3. Even with good intake, however, many factors suggest that diet alone cannot meet the total nutritional needs for some individuals. The next chapter offers information on vitamin and mineral supplementation.

Chapter Summary

Nutrition refers to the ingestion of foods and their relationship to human health. All humans require the same basic nutrients, although the amount and type can vary based on age, diseases, and special needs.

Changes to nutritional habits can begin with just a few new actions that are achievable. A food journal can be a useful tool for assessing nutritional status and could include what is eaten, time consumed, with whom, and the feelings associated with food consumption.

Six small meals, beginning with a good breakfast, provide a regularity of intake that helps maintain good energy. The Food Guide Pyramid, which promotes a diet high in plant foods and low in animal foods and fat, is a guide for the types of foods to include in the diet. When planning dietary intake, consideration should be given to the macronutrients, which include water, carbohydrates, protein, and fat, and the micronutrients, which consist of vitamins and minerals.

References

1. Nightingale, F. (1860). *Notes on Nursing*. New York: D. Appleton and Co.
2. Hahnemann, S. (1982). Organon of medicine. In Kunzli, J., Alain, N., & Pendleton, P. (eds.). *The First Integral English Translation of the Definitive Sixth Edition of the Original Work on Homoeopathic Medicine*. Blaine, Washington: Cooper Publishing, p. 110.
3. U.S. Department of Agriculture. (2008). Consumption of food away from home. Economics Research Service, Briefing Room. Retrieved August 1, 2008, from http://www.ers.usda.gov/Briefing/DietAndHealth/fafh.htm.

Suggested Readings

American Dietetic Association, & Duyff, R. L. (2006). *American Dietetic Association Complete Food and Nutrition Guide*. Hoboken, NJ: Wiley.

Atkins, R. C. (2003). *Atkins for Life: The Complete Controlled Carb Program for Weight Loss and Good Health*. New York: St. Martin's Press.

Balch, P. A. (2002). *Prescription for Nutritional Healing: The A-to-Z Guide to Supplements: The A-to-Z Guide to Supplements*. New York: Avery Press.

Balch, P. A., & Balch, J. F. (2000). *Prescription for Nutritional Healing*, 3rd ed. New York: Avery Press.

Balentine, R. (2007). *Diet and Nutrition: A Holistic Approach*. Honesdale, PA: Himalyan Press.

Macwilliam, L. (2007). *NutriSearch Comparative Guide to Nutritional Supplements*. Vernon, British Columbia, Canada: Northern Dimensions Publishing.

Mahan, K., & Escott-Stump, S. (2000). *Krause's Food, Nutrition, and Diet Therapy*, 10th ed. Philadelphia: W.B. Saunders.

PDR Staff. (2008). *2008 Physicians' Desk Reference (PDR) for Nonprescription Drugs, Dietary Supplements, and Herbs*, Montvale, NJ: Thomson.

U.S. Department of Agriculture and U.S. Department of Health and Human Services. (2005). *Nutrition and Your Health: Dietary Guidelines for Americans*, 6th ed. Washington, DC: U.S. Government Printing Office.

Wang, Y. C., Colditz, G. A., & Kuntz, K. M. (2007). Forecasting the obesity epidemic in the aging U.S. population. *Obesity*, 15(11):2855–2865.

Whitney, E. N., & Rolfes, S. R. (2007). *Understanding Nutrition*. New York: Wadsworth Press.

Willett, W. C. (2005). *Eat, Drink, and Be Healthy: The Harvard Medical School Guide to Healthy Eating*. New York: Fireside, Simon and Schuster.

Resources

American Diabetes Association
505 8th Ave.
New York, NY 10018
212-947-9707
www.diabetes.org

This Web site offers education, information, and referrals regarding diabetes.

The American Dietetic Association
216 West Jackson Blvd.
Chicago, IL 60606-6995
800-366-1655
Chicago Area: 312-899-0040
www.eatright.org/ncnd.html

This provides information about a variety of nutrition resources and programs and includes a "tip of the day," as well as numerous areas for reading.

American Heart Association
7320 Greenville Ave.
Dallas, TX 75231
214-750-5300
www.americanheart.org

This is an excellent site with areas called "Healthy Tools" and "Healthy Lifestyle," particularly geared to nutrition.

American Institute for Cancer Research
1759 R Street, NW
Washington, DC 20009
800-843-8114
Washington, DC Metropolitan area: 202-328-7744
www.aicr.org

This gives a variety of nutrition information relating to cancer.

Anorexia Nervosa and Related Eating Disorders
P.O. Box 5102
Eugene, OR 97405
503-344-1144
http://www.anred.com

This offers referrals and information on treatment of eating disorders.

Center for Science in the Public Interest
1875 Connecticut Ave., NW, Suite 300
Washington, DC 20009-5728
202-332-9110
www.cspinet.org/

The *Nutrition Action Healthletter* is an excellent source of nutrition information for just $15.00 per year. It offers quizzes on nutrition and health.

Food and Drug Administration Center for Food Safety and Applied Nutrition
1500 Paint Branch Parkway
College Park, MD 20740-3835
http://vm.cfsan.fda.gov

This is the FDA's Web site of the Center for Food Safety and Applied Nutrition. This provides information on food, food-borne illness, food labeling, food safety, special interest areas, and FDA documents; there are links to FDA home and other government sites.

Food and Nutrition Information Center, National Agricultural Library, Agricultural Research Service, USDA
10301 Baltimore Ave., Room 304
Beltsville, MD 20705-2351
www.nal.usda.gov/fnic

This resource offers a way to search any food-related topic on their Web site. Information on nutrition is given, along with links to other sites; it is updated daily.

International Food Information Council Publications Department, IFIC Foundation
1100 Connecticut Ave., NW, Suite 430
Washington, DC 20036
www.wheatfoods.org

This is devoted to help increase awareness of dietary grains as an essential component to a healthy diet.

Iowa State University, University Extension Food Science and Human Nutrition Extension
1127 Human Nutritional Sciences Bldg.
Iowa State University
Ames, IA 50011-1120
http://www.extension.iastate.edu/nutrition/

This user-friendly site is devoted entirely to nutrition and health with various calculators.

National Institute of Diabetes and Digestive and Kidney Diseases
Weight Control Information Network
1 WIN Way
Bethesda, MD 20892-3665
800-WIN-8098
www.niddk.nih.gov/health/nutrit/win.htm

This is a nicely laid out Web site that has information about nutrition and obesity.

National Women's Health Resource Center
2425 L Street, NW 3rd Floor
Washington, DC 20037
800-944-WOMAN (9662)
www.4woman.gov

US Department of Health and Human Services site offering information about women's health, nutrition, and many links to important resources.

Nutrient Data Laboratory USDA Agricultural Research Service
Beltsville Human Nutrition Research Center
4700 River Rd., Unit 89
Riverdale, MD 20737
301-734-8491
www.nal.usda.gov/fnic/foodcomp/

This USDA Nutrient Database gives facts about the composition of food, a glossary of terms, and links to other agencies.

Suburban Water Testing Labs
4600 Kutztown Rd.
Temple, PA 19560-1548
800-433-6595
http://www.h2otest.com/

This site sells water testing kits online; various kits test different problems.

Tufts University Health and Nutrition Letter
6 Beacon St., Suite 1110
Boston, MA 02108
617-557-4994
www.healthletter.tufts.edu/

This has an excellent subscription newsletter with a bonus for online subscribers, Web site rates, and links to other sites.

U.S. Department of Agriculture, Center for Nutrition Policy and Promotion
1120 20th Street, NW
Suite 200, North Lobby
Washington, DC 20036
202-418-2312
www.usda.gov/fcs/cnpp.htm

The Food Guide Pyramid and Dietary Guidelines can be downloaded by clicking the CNPP button from this Web site.

U.S. Department of Health and Human Services Consumer Information Center, Department WWW
P.O. Box 100
Pueblo, CO 81009
www.pueblo.gsa.gov/food.htm

Booklets on food and nutrition can be downloaded (free) or ordered through this site.

U.S. Food and Drug Administration, Center for Food Safety and Applied Nutrition
Food Labeling
5600 Fishers Ln. (HFE-88)
Room 1685
Rockville, MD 20847
301-443-9767
www.vm.cfsan.fda.gov/label.html

The *FDA Consumer Magazine* is accessible through this Web site, as well as a plethora of information about health, nutrition, and dietary choices.

University of Maryland, Cooperative Extension Service
Extension Publications On-Line
Publications Office
Symons Hall
University of Maryland at College Park
College Park, MD 20742
www.agnr.umd.edu/CES/Pubs/newsletters.html#nut

This Web site contains a summary of articles in recent editions of their extension publications. The nutrition button at this Web site will allow you to view nutrition articles with many interesting topics from weight control to Food Guide Pyramid choices.

University of Minnesota, Department of Food Science and Nutrition
Nutritionist's Tool Box
1334 Eckles Ave.
Saint Paul, MN 55108
612-624-1290
www.fsci.umn.edu/tools.htm

This site offers a calorie calculator and a nutrition analysis tool to analyze the foods you eat for a variety of nutrients.

Watersafe Test Kits
Silver Lake Research Corporation
P.O. Box 686
Monrovia, CA 91017
888-438-1942
www.watersafetestkits.com

This site offers water testing kits for sale and also provides information on buying their kits in retail stores.

Chapter 3

Dietary Supplements

OBJECTIVES

This chapter should enable you to

- Describe the difference between recommended daily allowances and dietary reference intakes
- Discuss the development of the nutritional supplement industry
- List factors to consider in assessing the need for supplements
- Describe facts that are listed on supplement labels
- List the antioxidants and their sources
- Define the term *phytochemical*
- Discuss health conditions for which nutritional supplements can be beneficial

The importance of proper and sensible nutrition, as stated in the previous chapter, cannot be emphasized enough. In its Healthy People 2010 Report, the U.S. Government's Office of Disease Prevention and Health Promotion states that what people eat, especially when they exercise regularly and do not smoke and/or drink excessively, is the most significant controllable risk factor affecting their long-term health.[1] Basic dietary principles supporting optimum health included the following:

- Eating a wide variety of foods that provide adequate nutrients, including plenty of fresh fruits and vegetables, complex carbohydrates, plant protein, and fiber
- Keeping consumption of sugary foods, caffeinated beverages, and alcohol to a minimum
- Eating only a small amount of animal protein and fat
- Drinking plenty of water

It was once thought that anyone who followed these principles was considered properly nourished and did not need supplementation; however, the dietary habits of most Americans lead them to be overweight and undernourished.

Views on Vitamin Supplementation

Much debate has been going on regarding vitamins and minerals as nutritional supplements and how (or if) they should be taken daily. The early 1900s focused largely on deficiencies of vitamins and minerals that caused diseases such as scurvy and beriberi. Vitamins began to be added to food—a process called fortification. Through the 1950s and 1960s, a growing number of foods were fortified, such as breads, cereals, and milk. The addition of calcium has been among the recent fortification of many food products.

By the mid 1970s, however, the focus was less on vitamin deficiency and more on the value of vitamin and mineral supplementation for the prevention of illness and disease. Vitamin C was thought to alleviate symptoms and prevent the common cold. Vitamin E was said to help keep the heart healthy. A low-fat, high-fiber diet was the order of the decade. The late 1970s saw the response of the U.S. Senate Select Committee on Nutrition that listed the number one public health problem in this country as poor nutrition. Experts believed Americans consumed too much food of too little nutritive value and that this was a contributing factor to poor quality of life and increased disease.[2]

KEY POINT

Over the past decade, there has been an explosion in the use of nutritional supplements, which has caused the government to begin to regulate the supplement industry.

How the Government Is Involved

Recommended Dietary Allowances

Since the 1940s, the Food and Nutrition Board of the National Academy of Sciences has made recommendations for nutrient intake. These recommendations have been termed recommended dietary allowances (RDAs) and represent the standards that should meet the needs of most healthy people in the United States. The RDAs address energy, protein, and most vitamins and minerals. Fats and carbohydrates standards were set in 2002[3]; they had never been set before that time because the experts assumed that if the average person met the energy requirements for protein then the demand for fats and carbohydrates would also be met.

There has been much confusion surrounding RDAs. Most consumers have had some misunderstanding of how to use RDAs and what food choices best meet these recommendations. The misconception exists that RDAs are optimum daily requirements rather than recommended minimum intakes as a standard for healthy individuals. The development of daily values (DV) and dietary reference intakes (DRIs) is phasing out RDAs.

> **KEY POINT**
>
> The RDAs reflect the minimum, not optimum, daily requirements for nutrients.

Dietary Reference Intakes

In an attempt to continue focusing on the benefits of healthy eating, DRIs were developed to update RDAs. These new guidelines represent the latest understanding of nutrient requirements for optimum health. The first set focused on nutrients related to bone health and fluoride[4]; in 1998, folate, the B vitamins, and choline were added.[5] Vitamin C, vitamin E, selenium, and carotenoids came in 2000[6]; in 2001 recommendations were published for vitamin A, vitamin K, arsenic, boron, chromium, copper, iodine, iron, manganese, molybdenum, nickel, silicon, vanadium, and zinc (micronutrients).[7] Additional nutrients and electrolytes are anticipated to be added in the future.

The need to update and change the standards for intake of nutrients remains a challenge. The Food and Nutrition Board of the National Academy of Sciences is updating these standards on a regular basis. The newest work through these agencies is called daily values (DVs). DVs are divided into two groups: reference daily intakes (RDIs) and daily reference values (DRVs). RDIs are to be used in reference to vitamins, minerals, and proteins.

DRIs are divided into four subcategories:

1. Estimated average requirements (EARs)[8]
2. RDAs, continued from 1989
3. Adequate intakes
4. Tolerable upper intake levels

EARs would satisfy 50% of requirements for men and women for specific age groups and are intended for use by nutritional professionals. If calculations of EARs are not available, adequate intakes are used instead of RDAs. RDAs continue to be considered as sufficient amounts of nutrients to meet nearly all needs. Tolerable upper intake levels indicate the largest amount of a nutrient that someone can ingest without adverse affect.[9]

> **KEY POINT**
>
> In 1994, an office was created within the National Institutes of Health (NIH) for overseeing research on dietary supplements through the Dietary Supplement Health and Education Act (DSHEA). This requires manufacturers to include the words *dietary supplement* on product labels.

The Food and Drug Administration (FDA) describes acceptable claims that can be made for relationships between a nutrient and the risk of a disease or health-related condition. These claims must be clear as to the relationship of the nutrient to the disease and be understandable by the general public. The claims can be made in several ways: through third-party references (such as the National Cancer Institute), symbols (such as a heart), and vignettes or descriptions (see Exhibit 3-1).

The FDA does not allow claims for healing, treatment, or cure of specific medical conditions on the labels or advertisements of nutritional supplements. This would put supplements in the category of drugs. The DSHEA allows only three types of claims to be used with supplements: nutrient content, disease, and nutrition support claims. The nutrient content explains how much of a nutrient is in a supplement. Claims regarding disease must have a basis in scientific evidence and refer to health-related conditions or diseases and a particular

---

EXHIBIT 3-1   Status of Health Claims

Approved Health Claims for Dietary Supplements and Conventional Foods

· Calcium and osteoporosis
· Folate and neural tube defects
· Soluble fiber from whole oats and coronary heart disease
· Soluble fiber from psyllium husks and coronary heart disease
· Sugar alcohols and dental caries

Approved Health Claims for Conventional Foods Only

· Dietary lipids and cancer
· Dietary saturated fat and cholesterol and coronary heart disease
· Fiber-containing grain products, fruits, and vegetables and cancer
  · Fruits and vegetables and cancer (for foods that are naturally a "good source" of vitamin A, vitamin C, or dietary fiber)
  · Fruits, vegetables, and grain products that contain fiber, particularly soluble fiber, and coronary heart disease
· Sodium and hypertension

Health Claims Not Authorized

· Antioxidant vitamins and cancer
· Dietary fiber and cancer
· Dietary fiber and cardiovascular disease
· Omega-3 fatty acids and coronary heart disease
· Zinc and immune function in older individuals

Source: The Commission on Dietary Supplementation

nutrient. Nutrition support claims (which may be used without FDA approval, but not without notification to that agency) are set up to explain how a deficiency could develop if the diet was deficient in that nutrient. These claims are accompanied by an FDA disclaimer on the label of the supplement and are therefore easy to determine. In March 1999, the DSHEA required that all nutritional supplements carry a "Supplement Facts" panel (see Figure 3-1).

Figure 3-1   Supplement Label

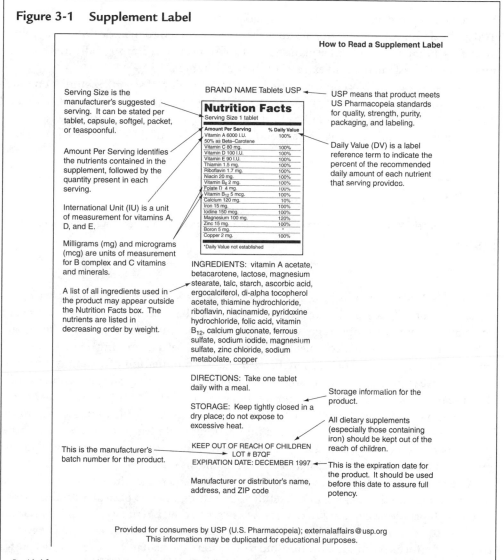

How to Read a Supplement Label

Serving Size is the manufacturer's suggested serving. It can be stated per tablet, capsule, softgel, packet, or teaspoonful.

Amount Per Serving identifies the nutrients contained in the supplement, followed by the quantity present in each serving.

International Unit (IU) is a unit of measurement for vitamins A, D, and E.

Milligrams (mg) and micrograms (mcg) are units of measurement for B complex and C vitamins and minerals.

A list of all ingredients used in the product may appear outside the Nutrition Facts box. The nutrients are listed in decreasing order by weight.

This is the manufacturer's batch number for the product.

BRAND NAME Tablets USP

USP means that product meets US Pharmacopeia standards for quality, strength, purity, packaging, and labeling.

Daily Value (DV) is a label reference term to indicate the percent of the recommended daily amount of each nutrient that serving provides.

Nutrition Facts
Serving Size 1 tablet

Amount Per Serving	% Daily Value
Vitamin A 6000 I.U.	100%
50% as Beta–Carotene	
Vitamin C 80 mg.	100%
Vitamin D 100 I.U.	100%
Vitamin E 90 I.U.	100%
Thiamin 1.5 mg.	100%
Riboflavin 1.7 mg.	100%
Niacin 20 mg.	100%
Vitamin B₆ 2 mg.	100%
Folate D .4 mg.	100%
Vitamin B₁₂ 5 mcg.	100%
Calcium 120 mg.	10%
Iron 15 mg.	100%
Iodine 150 mcg.	100%
Magnesium 100 mg.	120%
Zinc 15 mg.	100%
Boron 5 mg.	*
Copper 2 mg.	100%

*Daily Value not established

INGREDIENTS: vitamin A acetate, betacarotene, lactose, magnesium stearate, talc, starch, ascorbic acid, ergocalciferol, di-alpha tocopherol acetate, thiamine hydrochloride, riboflavin, niacinamide, pyridoxine hydrochloride, folic acid, vitamin B₁₂, calcium gluconate, ferrous sulfate, sodium iodide, magnesium sulfate, zinc chloride, sodium metabolate, copper

DIRECTIONS: Take one tablet daily with a meal.

STORAGE: Keep tightly closed in a dry place; do not expose to excessive heat.

KEEP OUT OF REACH OF CHILDREN
LOT # B7QF
EXPIRATION DATE: DECEMBER 1997

Manufacturer or distributor's name, address, and ZIP code

Storage information for the product.

All dietary supplements (especially those containing iron) should be kept out of the reach of children.

This is the expiration date for the product. It should be used before this date to assure full potency.

Provided for consumers by USP (U.S. Pharmacopeia); externalaffairs@usp.org
This information may be duplicated for educational purposes.

Provided for consumers by USP (U.S. Pharmacopeial) external affairs

A Supplement Extravaganza

Vitamins and minerals were what traditionally made up typical nutritional supplements. Today the definition of nutritional supplements is expanded to include "vitamins, minerals, herbs, botanicals, and other plant-derived substances; and amino acids, concentrates, metabolites, constituents, and extracts of these substances."[10]

Consumers can easily become confused by the burgeoning of scientific studies on nutrients, the immediate release of single studies relating to nutrition, diet, and health, and supplement advertisements that use health claims to increase sales. In many cases, one report contradicts another—what was good yesterday is harmful today.

KEY POINT

Approximately 40% of adults in the United States use nutritional supplementation on a regular basis.

The New Millennium was accompanied by buzzwords, such as antioxidants, phytochemicals, functional foods, and nutriceuticals. It is yet to be determined whether these new compounds deserve the onslaught of press, print, and manufacture they so readily receive. When a new study has been completed that suggests a benefit from a nutrient, it is released immediately. Americans rush to purchase the latest combination of vitamins, minerals, and nutritive supplements—spending billions of dollars on dietary supplements annually. Are the supplements worth taking, and are the claims made by manufacturers true? Nutritional supplements may be helpful, but they may also be harmful. Taking supplements without knowledge of their actions and interactions could lead to imbalances of other nutrients and, potentially, toxicity; however, if taken properly and with forethought, supplements can increase general health and ward off some diseases.

When making the decision to take nutritional supplements, evaluation of the information available should be done in a carefully planned manner as part of a total nutrition program. If people hear of studies that seem to relate to their circumstances, it is important for them to do some investigating on their own. Studies need to be assessed in the context they were performed and their relationship to a person's particular situation. Health professionals can assist individuals in understanding what studies reveal. In any case, taking a supplement based on what has been read or heard in the news does not guarantee that a given person will have the same outcome.

The nutritional supplement industry is still in its infancy and grows exponentially each day. There continues to be an increasing variety of supplements readily available, which can be bought over the Internet, by mail order, at supermarkets, in drug stores, and in other types of stores. Supplements are no longer the domain of natural food stores. The FDA regulates and oversees manufacturing, product information, and safety, and the Federal Trade Commission regulates advertising of supplements; however, decisions regarding whether supplements should be taken, in what form, and how much, still remain a personal choice.

There is increasing interest among Americans to use nutritional supplements for optimum health. Some experts are also indicating a definite need for supplementation as part of a nutritional plan. Relying solely on diet to meet the body's needs for vitamins and minerals is fast becoming a thing of the past. We no longer eat food picked fresh from the local garden and cooked within hours. Additionally, many food preparation practices decrease the nutritive value of food.

Vitamins and minerals play an important role in optimum health and in reducing the risk of chronic diseases. Is the diet a person is consuming, however, giving him or her enough nutrients and meeting individual needs? If so, then all that may be needed is a good quality multivitamin/mineral; however, if a person has poor nutritional habits, is under a great deal of stress, is pregnant or planning a pregnancy, or has a health problem, supplementation is a must. The supplements that are needed, how much of each, and for how long they need to be taken then becomes the issue. The research is promising, but for many nutrients, the results are still not definite.

KEY POINT

Supplements can never substitute for a healthy, sensible nutrition program where whole foods, containing hundreds of substances, working together synergistically, are consumed. Poor food choices and eating habits cannot be banished by supplementation.

Age, nutritional lifestyle, quality and quantity of food, gender, life stage, environment, family history, personal history, diet, exercise, and rest patterns should be considered in determining a person's need for nutritional supplementation.

As with all holistic approaches, knowledge, self-care, balance, and using what nature provides are the keys. Individual nutritional needs can be determined by looking at the responses made on your Nutritional Lifestyle Survey (see Chapter 1) and by considering several factors:

Age: The need for nutrient supplementation increases with age. There are some nutrients that are not absorbed as well as a person ages, even if they are consumed in good quantity. Older adults may be affected by poor lifelong nutrition habits, social isolation, and chronic diseases that require special diets or affect food intake. Children need a balanced diet, along with a good quality multivitamin and limited sweets and fats to promote their growth and development.

Chronic health problems: Some chronic conditions create special nutritional needs, whereas others produce symptoms that threaten a healthy nutritional status. If a person has a chronic health problem, is taking medication, and wants to take nutritional supplements, a thorough knowledge of drug–supplement interactions is necessary. Nurses and other health practitioners can help in this area.

Women: Women who are pregnant, planning to become pregnant, breastfeeding, menopausal, or postmenopausal need added nutrients and/or supplementation. Different supplements are needed for different life cycles. Within the past decade, the National Academy of Sciences has increased DRIs for folate and calcium for women.[11,12] These are of great import for women.

Lifestyle choices: Cigarette and alcohol use reduces the levels of certain nutrients and predisposes the body to diseases for which added protection is helpful. A stressful lifestyle can deplete nutrients. Deficiencies also can arise from the high consumption of caffeine and sugar.

If people presently take multivitamin/mineral supplements and believe that they may benefit from taking additional supplements, they should first examine the labels of their food and supplements. They need to check the DVs of each vitamin and mineral listed. They should be receiving at least 100% for all nutrients from all food and supplements. If they are lower than 100%, they first need to determine whether they can meet this need through a change in diet. If they cannot meet the requirements through diet, then supplements of specific nutrients may be necessary. If the DV is over 100% for some or all nutrients, they may want to cut back on that supplement. The guideline is to keep below 300% DV of any nutrient. A nutritional analysis can be used, also. A registered dietician, nutritionist, or nutrition-knowledgeable healthcare professional can help with an analysis. Some Web sites offer free nutritional analysis (see the resources section at the end of this chapter).

KEY POINT

When using supplements, always read the labels. Know what you are taking, how easily it is absorbed, if it has United States Pharmacopeia (USP) initials, and when it expires, and by all means, if you have any adverse affects—stop taking it.

Supplement Labels

Supplements come in many forms: tablets, capsules, softgels, powders, and liquids. The USP is the agency that oversees drug products and sets the standards for dietary supplements. All supplements now require labels, which are regulated by the USP. The USP has certain standards that must be met for single vitamins and those in combination, as well as dietary supplements, and botanical and herbal preparations. Figure 3-1 shows the information that is contained on a supplement label.

One facet of the dietary supplement label that is important to read is the DV column. The DV is the percentage of the recommended daily amount of the nutrient that a serving gives. According to the USP, intake should be between 50% and 100% of the DV of each nutrient. One nutrient that would not provide 100% of the DV is calcium. If 100% of calcium were added to any supplement, it would be too big to swallow. Calcium should be taken in divided doses throughout the day.

The bioavailability of a particular nutrient is the amount of a nutrient that enters the blood stream and actually reaches the various organs, tissues, and cells of the body. Nutrients have greater bioavailability when they are taken with compounds that help their absorption.

Fruits and vegetables contain many compounds that, when eaten, allow for synergy to take place in the body, increasing bioavailability. Fruits and vegetables are especially affected by mode of storage and preparation. Those that have been exposed to heat, light, or air have lost some or all of their nutrients; their bioavailability is lowered.

Two important factors when considering the bioavailability of a supplement are ease of absorption and the benefit of taking it in combination with another supplement. Disintegration (how quickly a tablet/supplement breaks apart) and dissolution (how fast the supplement dissolves in the intestinal tract)[13] are two additional factors directly related to bioavailability. Vitamin C assists with the absorption of iron into the body. If taking iron as a supplement, people also should consider their vitamin C intake. Taking an iron supplement with a glass of orange juice would increase the bioavailability of the iron. On the other hand, calcium inhibits iron and magnesium absorption. This is important to remember when adding supplements to a nutritional plan, especially if iron, calcium, and vitamin C individually or in a multivitamin are being taken. More research is needed to determine and document supplement interactions. The NIH recently issued a call for research, mandated by Congress, "to explore the current state of our knowledge about the important issues related to bioavailability of nutrients and other bioactive components from dietary supplements."[14]

Birth Defects

One of the first vitamins addressed by the advisory committee on dietary supplements was folic acid. The original aim was said to reduce neural tube birth defects, especially spina bifida. The RDA for folic acid was doubled from 200 to 400 mcg/day. The Centers for Disease Control, the USP, the FDA, and the March of Dimes have all recommended that women of childbearing age consume 400 mcg per day of folic acid, either through diet or supplements[15] (see Figure 3-2). Women who are planning to become pregnant and who are of childbearing age should eat a varied diet and also take folic acid through supplementa-

---

Figure 3-2 Folic Acid

Women and Folic Acid

Folic acid is a B vitamin that everyone needs to help cells grow and divide. It is especially important for women who may become pregnant.

Why is Folic Acid So Important for Women?

Taken before and during early pregnancy, folic acid, also known as folate, reduces the chances of having a baby born with birth defects of the spine and brain (spina bifida and anencephaly). If you have already had a baby with spina bifida or anencephaly, see your doctor if you are considering another pregnancy.

For women of childbearing years USP, the CDC, the FDA, and the March of Dimes all recommend 400 mcg of folic acid daily.

You should not take more than 1000 mcg daily unless your healthcare professional tells you to do so.

How Can I Get an Adequate Amount of Folic Acid?

It is possible to get folic acid by eating foods such as green leafy vegetables; cereal and cereal products; and citrus fruits and juices. Certain fully fortified breakfast cereals have 100% of the recommended daily amount of folic acid. Many women, however, prefer to take a multivitamin supplement.

What About a Dietary Supplement?

Folic acid may be taken as a tablet or as part of a multivitamin supplement. Make certain that the letters "USP" appear on the label to ensure that your vitamin/mineral product meets established standards for strength, quality, and purity.

Where Can I Find Additional Information About Pregnancy and Folic Acid?

Centers for Disease Control and Prevention
Mail Stop F 45
4770 Buford Highway N.E.
Atlanta, GA 30341-3724
770/488-7160
e-mail: pgm5@cdc.gov

Food and Drug Administration
HFE-88
5600 Fishers Lane
Rockville, MD 20857
800/332-4010
http://www.fda.gov

March of Dimes
1275 Mamaroneck Avenue
White Plains, NY 10605
888/663-4637
e-mail: resourcecenter@modimes.org

Spina Bifida Association of America
4590 MacArthur Blvd.
Suite 250
Washington, D.C. 20007
202/944-3285
e-mail: sbaa@sbaa.org

United States Pharmacopeia
12601 Twinbrook Parkway
Rockville, MD 20852
301/816-8223
e-mail: externalaffairs@usp.org

*Ask your healthcare professional
to help you determine your need for
folic acid supplements.*

Provided for consumers by USP (U.S. Pharmacopeia); externalaffairs@usp.org
This information may be duplicated for educational purposes.

tion. Sufficient folate is critical from conception through the first four to six weeks of pregnancy when the neural tube is formed. This means adequate diet and supplement use should begin well before pregnancy occurs.

KEY POINT

The neural tube is a type of membrane that grows into the spinal cord and brain in utero (during pregnancy). Neural tube defects are problems in the development of the brain and spinal cord that arise during pregnancy. This is now believed to be a result of folate deficiency of the mother in the weeks before and in the early weeks of pregnancy. It is estimated that nearly 50% of all neural tube defects that occur can be arrested by adequate folate intake.

Antioxidants

Antioxidants are compounds that naturally protect the body from free radicals and help to depress the effects of metabolic by-products that cause degenerative changes related to aging. Mounting evidence shows that antioxidants play a role in preventing or delaying the onset of diseases such as cancer, stroke, arthritis, heart disease, immune problems, and neurological problems.[16]

Free radicals have a helpful function in the body, but in higher levels, they can damage cells and tissues. They are produced by the body's own metabolism and are generated from exposure to environmental factors and toxins. Antioxidant nutrients are said to neutralize the harmful free radicals that occur in the body constantly and arise from improper nutrition, eating fatty foods; smoking; drinking alcohol; taking drugs; and exposure to environmental pollutants (such as herbicides and pesticides), toxins, carcinogens, iron, smog, and radiation.

The body has natural antioxidant enzymes that regulate the effects of free radicals. These enzymes are catalase, superoxide dismutase, and glutathione peroxidase. Vitamins A (as beta-carotene), C, and E, and selenium assist the enzymes in the body to fight free radical damage.

Benefits Versus Risks of Antioxidant Supplementation

A diet low in fats, sweets, and animal protein that includes at least five fruits and vegetables per day, in variety, is a much safer way to obtain antioxidant protection than through supplementation. A greater chance of imbalances and toxicity exists when supplements are being used (Tables 3-1 and 3-2 show guidelines for information on vitamins and minerals); however, there continues to be increased evidence supporting antioxidant supplements as part of nutritional lifestyle.

TABLE 3-1 Vitamins

Vitamin	Deficiency may cause	How it works
A	Night blindness, skin problems, dry inflamed eyes	Bone and teeth growth, vision, keeps cells, skin, and tissues working properly
B-1 Thiamin	Tiredness, weakness, loss of appetite, emotional upset, nerve damage to legs (late sign)	Helps release food nutrients and energy, appetite control, helps nervous system, and digestive tract
B-2 Riboflavin	Cracks at corners of mouth, sensitivity to light, eye problems, inflamed mouth	Helps enzymes in releasing energy from cells, promotes growth, cell oxidation
Niacin	General fatigue, digestive disorders, irritability, loss of appetite, skin disorders	Fat, carbohydrate, and protein metabolism, good skin, tongue & digestive system, circulation
B-6 Pyridoxine	Dermatitis, weakness, convulsions in infants, insomnia, poor immune response, sore tongue, confusion, irritability	Necessary protein metabolism, nervous system functions, formation of red blood cells, immune system function
Biotin	Rarely seen since it can be made in body if not consumed. Flaky skin, loss of appetite, nausea.	Cofactor with enzymes for metabolism of macronutrients, formation of fatty acids, helps other B vitamins be utilized
Folic Acid	Anemia, diarrhea, digestive upset, bleeding gums,	red blood cell formation, healthy pregnancy, metabolism of proteins
B12 Cobalamin	Elderly, vegetarians, or those with malabsorption disorder are at risk of deficiency-pernicious anemia, nerve damage	Necessary to form blood cells, proper nerve function, metabolism of carbohydrates and fats, builds genetic material
Pantothenic Acid	Not usually seen; vomiting, cramps, diarrhea, fatigue, tingling hands and feet, difficult coordination	Needed for many processes in body, converts nutrients into energy, formation of some fats, vitamin utilization, making hormones

Excess may cause	Best foods to eat
Birth defects, bone fragility, vision and liver problems	Eggs, dark green and deep orange fruits and vegetables, liver, whole milk
Headache, rapid pulse irritability, trembling, insomnia, interference, with B2, B6	Whole grains and enriched breads, cereals, dried beans, pork, most vegetables, nuts, peas
No known toxic effect Some antibiotics can interfere with B2 being absorbed	Whole grains, enriched bread & cereals, leafy, green vegetables, dairy, eggs, yogurt
Flushing, stomach pain, nausea, eye damage, can lead to heart and liver damage	Whole wheat, poultry, milk, cheese, nuts, potatoes, tuna, eggs
Reversible nerve injury, difficulty walking, numbness, impaired senses	Wheat and rice bran, fish, lean meats, whole grains, sunflower seeds, corn, spinach, bananas
Symptoms similar to vitamin B1 overdose	Egg yolks, organ meats, vegetables, fish, nuts, seeds, also made in intestine by normal bacteria there
Excessive intake can mask B12 deficiency and interfere with zinc absorption	Green leafy vegetables, organ meats, dried beans
None known except those born with defect to absorb	Liver, salmon, fish, lean meats, milk, all animal products
Rare	Lean meats, whole grains, legumes

(continues)

TABLE 3-1 **Vitamins** *(continued)*

Vitamin	Deficiency may cause	How it works
C Ascorbic Acid	Bleeding gums, slow healing, poor immune response, aching joints, nose bleeds, anemia	Helps heal wounds, collagen maintenance, resistance to infection, formation of brain chemicals
D	Poor bone growth, rickets, osteoporosis, bone softening, muscle twitches	Calcium and phosphorus metabolism and absorption, bone and teeth formation
E	Not usually seen, after prolonged impairment of fat absorption, neurological abnormalities	Maintains cell membranes, assists as antioxidant, red blood cell formation
K	Tendency to hemorrhage, liver damage	Needed for prothrombin, blood clotting, works with Vitamin D in bone growth

Vitamin A

Vitamin A is necessary for good immune function, tissue repair, healthy skin and hair, bone formation, and vision. Fat-soluble vitamin A can cause toxicity and even be fatal in amounts higher than 10,000 IUs per day. There may be greater risk of birth defects for babies whose mothers take preformed vitamin A during pregnancy—especially during the first trimester.[17]

Beta-carotene, one of the family of carotenoids and a precursor to vitamin A, is a natural antioxidant, which enhances the immune system and may protect against certain cancers, cataracts, and heart disease. Beta-carotene is converted in the intestines and liver into preformed vitamin A; its sources are bright, orange-yellow fruits and vegetables.

Lycopene is another carotenoid and powerful antioxidant shown to reduce the risk of prostate and other cancers. The sources are fruits and vegetables of deep red to pink color. Some orange fruits and vegetables, some green leafy vegetables, and broccoli contain lutein, another carotenoid that has been found to arrest the development of macular degeneration and help protect the eyes from other diseases.[18]

Vitamin C

Vitamin C is a popular supplement often consumed in large amounts. Recent research may be causing consumers of this supplement to rethink their intake. Between 100 and 200 mg

Excess may cause	Best foods to eat
Diarrhea, kidney stones, blood problems, urinary problems	Most fruits, especially citrus fruits, melon, berries, and vegetables
Headache, fragile bones, high blood pressure, increased cholesterol, calcium deposits	Egg yolks, organ meats, fortified milk, also made in skin when exposed to sun
	Vegetable oils and margarine, wheat germ, nuts, dark green vegetables, whole grains
Jaundice (yellow skin) with synthetic form, flushing and sweating	Green vegetables, oats, rye, dairy, made in intestinal tract

of vitamin C is considered an optimum dose.[19] High doses can easily upset bowel function, causing diarrhea. The dose for each person is highly individualized. Dr. Andrew Weil suggests a trial-and-error method for finding your optimum dose, which he recommends to be 3000 to 6000 mg per day.[20] It is easy to have a 500-mg intake from eating at least six fruits and vegetables a day.

Vitamin E and Selenium

Vitamin E, discovered in the early 1920s, has antioxidant proprieties. It has been shown to decrease the risk of cardiovascular disease and some cancers and may offer protection from Parkinson's disease and slow the progression of Alzheimer's disease.

Vitamin E together with selenium offers powerful antioxidant properties. Selenium has anticancer properties. Plants grown in selenium-rich soil are the best source. Vitamin E and selenium has been found to reduce some cancers by 37%, and research has shown that the death rate from cancer was reduced by 50% in groups that took selenium supplements.[21]

Vitamin E comes in two forms: natural and synthetic. The natural type is preferred and usually is listed on the label as d-alpha tocopherol (d-alpha tocopheryl) acetate. Synthetic vitamin E is listed on the label as dl-alpha tocopherol (tocopheryl) acetate.

There is little evidence of vitamin E toxicity, but at high levels, it can increase the effect of anticoagulant (blood thinning) medications and may also interfere with vitamin K's action in the body (blood clotting).

TABLE 3-2 Minerals

Minerals	Deficiency may cause	How it works
Calcium	Rickets, soft bones, osteoporosis, cramps, numbness and tingling of arms and legs	Strong bones, teeth, muscle and nerve function, blood clotting
Phosphorus	Weakness and bone pain, otherwise rare	Works with calcium, helps with nerve, muscle, and heart function
Magnesium	Muscle weakness twitching, cardiac problems, tremors, confusion, formation of blood clots,	Needed for other minerals and enzymes to work, helps bone growth, muscle contraction
Potassium	Lethargy, weakness, abnormal heart rhythm, nervous disorders	Fluid balance, controls heart, muscle, nerve and digestive function
Iron	Anemia, weakness, fatigue, pallor, poor immune response	Forms of hemoglobin and myoglobin-supplies oxygen to cells muscles
Iodine	Goiter, weight gain, increased risk of breast cancer	Helps metabolize fat, thyroid function
Zinc	Poor growth, poor wound healing, loss of taste, poor sexual development	Works with many enzymes for metabolism and digestion, immune support, wound healing, reproductive development
Manganese	Nerve damage, dizziness, hearing problems	Enzyme cofactor for metabolism, controls blood sugar, nervous and immune functions
Copper	Rare, but can cause anemia and growth problems in children	Enzyme activation, skin pigment, needed to form nerve and muscle fibers, red blood cells
Chromium	Impaired glucose tolerance in low blood sugar and diabetes	Glucose metabolism
Selenium	Heart muscle abnormalities, infections, digestive disturbances	Antioxidant with vitamin E, protects against cancer, helps maintain healthy heart
Molybdenium	Unknown	Element of enzymes needed for metabolism. Helps store iron.

Excess may cause	Best foods to eat
Confusion, lethargy, blocks iron absorption, deposits in body	Dairy, salmon and small bony fish, tofu
Proper balance needed with calcium	Meat, poultry, fish, eggs, dairy, dried beans, whole grains
Proper balance needed with calcium, phosphorus, and vitamin D	Nuts, soybeans, dried beans, green vegetables
Vomiting, muscle weakness	Vegetables, fruits, dried beans, milk
Increased need for antioxidants, heart disorders	Red meats, fish, poultry, dried beans, eggs, leafy vegetables
Thyroid decreased activity, enlargement	Seafood, iodized salt, kelp, lima beans
Digestive problems, fever, dizziness, anemia, kidney problems	Lean meats, fish, poultry, yogurt
High doses affect iron absorption	Nuts, whole grains, avocados
Usually by taking supplements. Liver problems, diarrhea.	Nuts, organ meats, seafood
Most Americans have low intake	Brewer's yeast, whole grains, peanuts, clams
Nail, hair, and digestive problems, fatigue, garlic odor of breath	Meat and grains, dependent on soil in which they were raised
Gout, joint pains, copper deficiency	Beans, grains, peas, dark green vegetables

Vitamin E has been shown to help immune response, keep low-density lipoprotein cholesterol levels in check, and assist other antioxidants to be more available for use against free radicals. A diet that includes whole grains, wheat germ, nuts, sunflower oil, and corn oil will meet vitamin E RDAs. If you wish to consume 400 to 800 IUs per day, supplementation is necessary.

Phytochemicals

Phytochemicals (plant chemicals) are compounds that exist naturally in all plant foods and give them their color, flavor, and scent. They are the non-nutritive substances of plants and are not vitamins or minerals; nevertheless, phytochemicals have been associated with assisting the immune system, working as antioxidants, and fighting cancer.[22] Foods that have been identified as having these health benefits are fruits, vegetables, legumes, grains, seeds, soy, licorice, and green tea. Researchers have discovered many classes of phytochemicals in food. Isoflavones (phytoestrogens) and lignins (soy), lycopene (tomato), anthocyanins and proanthocyanidins (grapes, blueberries, cherries, and other red crops), saponins (whole grains and legumes), flavonoids (cherries, tea, and parsley), and isothiocyanates and indoles (broccoli, cauliflower, and cabbage), have antioxidant properties that may lower LDL (bad cholesterol levels) and curb growth of tumors.[23]

One example of a vegetable that has gotten much press over the last several years is broccoli. Broccoli is in the cruciferous family, which includes cauliflower, cabbage, kale, brussel sprouts, bok choy, and Swiss chard. Cruciferous vegetables are excellent sources of fiber, beta-carotene, vitamin C, and other vitamins and minerals. Their cross-shaped flowers give them their name. The phytochemicals that have been found in these vegetables are indoles, isothiocyanates, and sulforaphane, which assist the body in triggering the formation of enzymes that block hormones and may protect cells against damage from certain carcinogens. Research is promising with regard to these and other phytochemicals and cancer; however, more studies are needed.

Benefits and Risks of Phytonutrient Supplementation

The benefits of soy products have been clearly established in studies showing that soy fights cancer and lowers cholesterol levels; however, the use of soy products, especially in women who are vegetarians, has been linked to iron deficiency. One reason cited is that a vegetarian diet uses soy to replace the meat of conventional diets; therefore, supplementing the diet with vitamin C to enhance iron absorption is recommended.[24]

Optimum levels for phytochemicals have not yet been determined. Individual foods contain different phytochemicals in varying amounts, and experts believe that it is the combination of these compounds that may make the difference. Some scientists believe there are thousands of phytochemicals in a single food. Because researchers have advanced the most active phytonutrients found in fruits and vegetables over the last few years, it was inevitable that these components, in supplement form, would soon follow.

Although this provides an extremely convenient way of receiving the benefits of phytonutrients, supplements contain only isolated components and not the entire compound as it is found in the whole food state. Currently, it would be best to consume phytochemicals by eating a variety of fruits, vegetables, grains, and legumes. Supplementation with isolated phytochemicals is discouraged until more information is obtained.

Cardiovascular Health

Heart disease is the number one killer of Americans, although it is largely preventable. The main issue leading to cardiovascular problems is arteriosclerosis (buildup of fatty deposits on the inner wall of arteries) more commonly known as hardening of the arteries. There has been a preponderance of literature explaining many factors affecting a person's risk of heart disease. Some factors include diet, stress, heredity, and lifestyle. Over the last several years, researchers have indicated the important role that some B vitamins—especially B_6, B_{12}, and folic acid—play in cardiovascular health by lowering blood levels of homocysteine.

Homocysteine, an amino acid, forms in the blood vessels and can accumulate there as a result of the breakdown of protein in foods (such as meats and dairy). High levels of homocysteine may be a leading cause of atherosclerosis. Second, research shows that people over the age of 50 have been found to have lower levels of vitamin B_{12}. Although older adults may get sufficient vitamin B_{12} in their food, between 10–30% no longer have the ability to adequately absorb the naturally occurring form of B_{12}; therefore, the National Academies of Science recommends those over age fifty should consume foods fortified with B_{12} and add supplements if necessary.[25] B vitamins often work synergistically with each other as well as with other body processes, such as enzymes being activated; B vitamins in combination are the best way to supplement (see Exhibit 3-2).

EXHIBIT 3-2   Risks with Vitamin B Group Supplementation

There are risks associated with excess doses of certain vitamin B group vitamins, particularly niacin, B_6, folate, and choline. Vitamin B_6, when taken in amounts in excess of 100 mg per day can cause neuropathy (a disorder of the nerves), which could lead to weakness, pain, and numbness of the limbs. Niacin's upper level intake is 35 mg per day. Symptoms of overdose with niacin include flushing, itching, and warm sensation. The folate upper level limit is set at 1000 mcg (1 mg), whereas choline is set at 3.5 grams per day. Excess choline may lead to low blood pressure.

Thiamine, riboflavin, B_{12}, pantothenic acid, and biotin do not have upper limits set because of the lack of evidence suggesting adverse effects from high intakes of these B vitamins; however, excessive consumption of these B vitamins is not wise.

Vitamin A, as beta-carotene, vitamin C, calcium, magnesium, selenium, vitamin E, manganese, potassium, bioflavonoids, choline, and essential fatty acids (EFAs) are some nutrients that also have been linked to optimum cardiovascular health. These nutrients are needed to repair, protect, and prevent degeneration of the blood vessels.

Hypertension

High blood pressure responds very well to lifestyle changes. Increased fiber, low sodium intake, relaxation techniques, and exercise are helpful in lowering and maintaining blood pressure. The DASH diet (see Figure 3-3) suggests foods that tend to be rich in potassium, magnesium, and calcium; these are the minerals experts believe to be important for controlling blood pressure. Foods rich in potassium include bananas, apricots, grapes, oranges, spinach, lentils, and almonds.

When diuretics (fluid pills) are used, the addition of magnesium as a supplement may be needed. Diuretics cause fluid loss and when fluid is lost from the body it takes potassium and magnesium with it. Magnesium assists potassium to keep blood pressure levels optimum.

Diabetes Mellitus

Diabetes is a chronic disease that is one of the major causes of blindness in the United States. It is caused from either a defect in or insufficiency of insulin that does not allow for the management of appropriate blood glucose levels.

Food is broken down and absorbed by the body when you eat. *Enzymes*—chemicals made by the body with the help of nutrients—turn protein into amino acids and starches and sugars into their simple sugars. Fats are broken down into fatty acids. After this happens, there is usually a rise in blood sugar, leading to the hormone insulin being secreted by the pancreas (a gland located behind the stomach). Insulin assists in the movement of nutrients from the bloodstream into the muscles and fat tissues and also the liver. This allows the liver to stop producing glucose (blood sugar). If there is not enough insulin being excreted or if what is excreted is unable to be used, then diabetes develops.

Chromium was first found to have a relationship with insulin control in the body in the mid 1950s, and in the late 1970s, it was finally accepted as a nutrient. Chromium is a mineral, essential to the body, which acts cooperatively with other substances that control metabolism. It is a component of the glucose tolerance factor used to help with fat metabolism by transporting glucose to the cells (and being metabolized to produce energy) and activates certain enzymes. The recommended daily allowance of chromium is 50 to 200 mcg. It is believed that only 10% of the population of the United States receives enough chromium in their diet. Deficiency or inadequacy of chromium effectively blocks insulin function, resulting in elevated glucose levels. Supplementation decreases fasting glucose levels and insulin levels, improves glucose tolerance, and suppresses cholesterol and triglyceride levels.

Figure 3-3   The Dash Diet

Following The DASH Diet

The DASH eating plan shown below is based on 2000 calories a day. The number of daily servings in a food group may vary from those listed, depending on your caloric needs.

Use this chart to help plan your menus, or take it with you when you go to the store.

Food group	Daily servings (except as noted)	Serving sizes	Examples and notes	Significance of each food group to the DASH eating plan
Grains and grain products	7–8	1 slice bread ¹/₂ cup dry cereal* ¹/₂ cup cooked rice, pasta, or cereal	whole-wheat bread, English muffin, pita bread, bagel, cereals, grits, oatmeal, crackers, unsalted pretzels, popcorn	major sources of energy and fiber
Vegetables	4–5	1 cup raw leafy vegetable ¹/₂ cup cooked vegetable 6 oz vegetable juice	tomatoes, potatoes, carrots, green peas, squash, broccoli, turnip greens, collards, kale, spinach, artichokes, green beans, lima beans, sweet potatoes	rich sources of potassium, magnesium, and fiber
Fruits	4–5	6 oz fruit juice 1 medium fruit ¹/₄ cup dried fruit ¹/₂ cup fresh, frozen, or canned fruit	apricots, bananas, dates, grapes, oranges, orange juice, grapefruit, grapefruit juice, mangoes, melons, peaches, pineapples, prunes, raisins, strawberries, tangerines	important sources of potassium, magnesium, and fiber
Low-fat or fat-free dairy foods	2–3	8 oz milk 1 cup yogurt 1 ¹/₂ oz cheese	fat-free (skim) or low-fat (1%) milk, fat-free or low-fat buttermilk, fat-free or low-fat regular or frozen yogurt, low-fat and fat-free cheese	major sources of calcium and protein
Meats, poultry, and fish	2 or less	3 oz cooked meats, poultry, or fish	select only lean; trim away visible fats; broil, roast, or boil, instead of frying; remove skin from poultry	rich sources of protein and magnesium
Nuts, seeds, and dry beans	4–5 per week	¹/₃ cup or 1 ¹/₂ oz nuts 2 tbsps or ¹/₂ oz seeds ¹/₂ cup cooked dry beans	almonds, filberts, mixed nuts, peanuts, walnuts, sunflower seeds, kidney beans, lentils, and peas	rich sources of energy, magnesium, potassium, protein, and fiber
Fats and oils**	2–3	1 tsp soft margarine 1 tbsp low-fat mayonnaise 2 tbsps light salad dressing 1 tsp vegetable oil	soft margarine, low-fat mayonnaise, light salad dressing, vegetable oil (such as olive, corn, canola, or safflower)	besides watching fats added to foods, choose foods that contain less fat
Sweets	5 per week	1 tbsp sugar 1 tbsp jelly or jam 1/2 oz jelly beans 8 oz lemonade	maple syrup, sugar, jelly, jam, fruit-flavored gelatin, jelly beans, hard candy, fruit punch, sorbet, ices	sweets should be low in fat

* Serving sizes vary between ¹/₂ and 1 ¹/₄ cups. Check the product's nutrition label.
** Fat content changes the serving sizes for fats and oils. For example, 1 tbsp of regular salad dressing equals 1 serving; 1 tbsp of a low-fat dressing equals ¹/₂ serving; 1 tbsp of a fat-free dressing equals 0 servings.

DASH

Essential Fatty Acids

The two essential fatty acids necessary for life and the proper function of the body are omega-3 (alpha-linoleic) and omega-6 (linoleic). EFAs enhance immune function, protect the lining of the gastrointestinal system, increase kidney blood flow, reduce inflammation, and inhibit platelet aggregation (cells of the blood sticking together). These fatty acids become converted with the help of enzymes eicosanoids. Prostaglandins are probably the most commonly known eicosanoids. One to two tablespoons of flaxseed ground fresh and sprinkled on food will provide an adequate amount of omega-3 oil for the average person. Cold-pressed and fresh canola, sunflower, an safflower oils are excellent sources of EFAs. These can be easily incorporated into your daily nutritional plan. Supplementation should be considered if a person has a health problem or does not include these nutrients in the diet.

KEY POINT

Omega-3 oils are found in fish oils and flaxseed; the omega-6 oil sources are borage (an herb), evening primrose, and black currant oils.

Osteoporosis

Calcium is an important mineral and may help prevent osteoporosis. When bones are calcium-rich, they are less susceptible to fractures. The new DRIs suggest that Americans take between 1000 and 1300 mg of calcium per day. After menopause, some women may require up to 1500 mg of calcium per day. The upper tolerable limit for calcium is set at 2500 mg per day. Excess calcium can cause muscle cramps, kidney stones, high blood calcium, or poor absorption of iron, zinc, or magnesium.

When considering calcium intake, it is important to know that vitamin D is essential in metabolizing and absorbing the calcium that you are ingesting. Magnesium and phosphorus are minerals that work together with calcium. Meeting calcium requirements means consuming adequate supplies of calcium and vitamin D. If people depend on dietary sources for these nutrients they may have to eat a very large quantity of calcium-rich foods in addition to consuming foods that include vitamin D, phosphorus, and magnesium in the proper ratios. There are several forms of calcium available in supplements; the most bioavailable form is calcium citrate; the least absorbable is calcium carbonate.

Sorting It All Out

The concept that people must be constantly on guard and change course to follow the most recent scientific study, not really knowing if they are heading in the right direction, is ominous. Nutritional supplementation can seem like a daunting task and quickly becomes overwhelming, unless the basics are implemented. Rather than becoming overloaded with facts regarding optimum nutritional supplementation, people should focus on eating basic, well-balanced diets. When a balanced diet is eaten, many compounds are consumed that help with the protection, breakdown, absorption, and integration of all that is ingested. Nature provides what is needed with the proper ingredients in the right amounts for the body—if a nutritious and healthful food plan is followed. If people are confused or have any doubt regarding what or how much they should be taking, consulting a healthcare practitioner who is knowledgeable in nutrition and nutrition supplementation for guidance is beneficial.

Summary

RDAs represent minimum standards of food intake to meet the needs of an average person, whereas DRIs go beyond RDAs to describe nutrient requirements for optimal health.

In 1994, the Dietary Supplement Health and Education Act required manufacturers to include the words dietary supplement on product labels and established an oversight office within the NIH.

It is important to read supplement labels. Factors to consider when contemplating the use of supplements include age, the presence of chronic health problems, gender, and lifestyle habits. Supplements can never replace a healthy diet.

Antioxidants include vitamins A, C, E, and selenium. Phytochemicals are compounds that exist naturally in all plant foods.

Supplements can be beneficial in the treatment of many chronic conditions; however, they must be used wisely. People need to learn about the actions, interactions, and risks associated with the specific supplements they use.

References

1. U.S. Department of Health and Human Services, Office of Disease Prevention and Health Promotion Healthy People 2010. Available from http://www.healthypeople.gov/
2. U.S. Senate (the McGovern Report) Select Committee on Nutrition and Human Needs. (1977). *Dietary Goals for the U.S.*, 2nd ed. Washington, DC: U.S. Government Printing Office.
3. National Academies of Science. (2002). *New Eating and Physical Activity Targets to Reduce Chronic Disease Risk*. National Academies of Science Press Release, September 5, 2002.
4. National Academies of Science. (2004). Dietary Reference Intakes (DRIs). Retrieved January 1, 2008, from http://www.iom.edu/Object.File/Master/21/372/0.pdf
5. National Academies of Science. (1998). *Dietary Reference Intakes for Thiamin, Riboflavin, Niacin, Vitamin B6, Folate, Vitamin B12, Pantothenic Acid, Biotin, and Choline*. National Academy of Science Press Release, April 7, 1998.
6. National Academies of Science. (2001). *Antioxidants' Role in Chronic Disease Prevention Still Uncertain; Huge Doses Considered Risky*. National Academy of Sciences Press Release, April 10, 2000.
7. Russell, R. (2001, January 9). *Dietary Reference Intakes for Vitamin A, Vitamin K, Arsenic, Boron, Chromium, Copper, Iodine, Iron, Manganese, Molybdenum, Nickel, Silicon, Vanadium, and Zinc*. Opening Statement, Institute of Medicine, Public Briefing, Washington, DC.
8. Institute of Medicine. Dietary Reference Intakes. Retrieved January 10, 2008, from http://www.iom.edu/CMS/3788/4574.aspx

9. National Academies of Science. (2004). *A Report of the Panel of Micronutrient, Subcommittee on Upper Reference Levels of Nutrients and of Interpretations and Uses of Dietary Reference Intakes, and the Standing Committee on Scientific Evaluation of Dietary Reference Intakes.* Washington, DC: Food and Nutrition Board, IOM, and National Academy of Sciences Press. Retrieved from http://www.iom.edu/Object.File/Master/21/372/0.pdf

10. *What Are Dietary Supplements?* National Institutes of Health, Office of Dietary Supplements Web site. Retrieved August 10, 2003, from www.ods.od.nih.gov

11. Eldridge, A. L. (2004). Comparison of 1989 RDAs and DRIs for water-soluble vitamins. *Nutrition Today. 39*(2):88–93.

12. Barr, S. I., Murphy, S. P., & Poos, M. I., (2002). Interpreting and using the Dietary Reference Intakes in dietary assessment of individuals and groups. *Journal of the American Dietetic Association, 102*:6.

13. United States Pharmacopeia. (2008). Dietary Supplements Lexicon. Retrieved August 1, 2008, from www.usp.org

14. Scalli, S., Zaid, A., & Soulamaymani, R. (2007). Drug interactions with herbal medicines. *Therapeutic Drug Monitor. 29*(6):679–686.

15. Centers for Disease Control and Prevention. (2008). Folic Acid. PHS Recommendations. Retrieved August 4, 2008 from http://www.cdc.gov/ncbddd/folicacid/health_recomm.htm

16. Rahman, K. (2007). Studies on free radicals, antioxidants, and co-factors. *Clinical Interventions in Aging. 2*(2):219–236.

17. Strobel, M., Tinz, J., & Bielsalski, H. K. (2007). The importance of beta-carotene as a source of vitamin A with special regard to pregnant and breastfeeding women. *European Journal of Nutrition. 2007*(46 Suppl 1):I1–I20.

18. VERIS. (2002). *Carotenoids and Eye Health.* LaGrange, IL: VERIS Research Information Services.

19. Levine, M. Wang, Y., Padayatty, S. & & Morrow, J. (2001, August 14). New Recommendations for Vitamin C. *Proceedings of the National Academy of Sciences, 98*:9842–9846.

20. Weil, A. (2006). *8 Weeks to Optimum Health: A Proven Program for Taking Full Advantage of Your Body's Natural Healing Power.* New York: Alfred A. Knopf Publishers, p. 57.

21. Peters, U., Littman, A. J., Kristal, A. R., Patterson, R. E., Potter, J. D., & White, E. (2007). Vitamin E and selenium supplementation and risk of prostate cancer in the Vitamins and lifestyle (VITAL) study cohort. *Cancer Causes and Control. 18*(8):1131–40.

22. Beliveau, R., & Gingras, D. (2007). Role of nutrition in preventing cancer. *Canadian Family Physician, 53*(11):1905–1911.

23. Johnson, I. T. (2007). Phytochemicals and cancer. *Proceedings of the Nutrition Society, 66*(2):207–215.

24. Venderley, A. M., & Campbell, W. W. (2006). Vegetarian diets : nutritional considerations for athletes. *Sports Medicine, 36*(4):293–305.

25. Food and Nutrition Board, National Institutes of Medicine. (2008). Dietary Reference Intakes: A Risk Assessment Model for Establishing Upper Intake Levels for Nutrients. Retrieved August 1, 2008 from http://www.nap.edu/catalog.php?record_id=6432#toc

Suggested Reading

Balentine, R. (2007). *Diet and Nutrition: A Holistic Approach.* Honesdale, PA: Himalyan Press.

Igloe, R. S., & Hui, Y. H. (2001). *Dictionary of Food Ingredients*, 4th ed. New York: Chapman and Hall.

Lieberman, S., & Bruning, N. P. (2003). *The Real Vitamin and Mineral Book.* New York: Penguin.

MacWilliam, L. (2007). *Comparative Guide to Nutritional Supplements*, 3rd ed. Oswego, NY: Northern Dimensions Publishing.

Mindell, E. (2004). *Earl Mindell's Vitamin Bible for the 21st Century*. New York: Time Warner Books.

Murray, M. (1998). *Encyclopedia of Nutritional Supplements*, 2nd ed. Rocklin, CA: Prima Publishing.

PDR Staff. (2008). *PDR for Nonprescription Drugs, Dietary Supplements, and Herbs, 2008 Physicians' Desk Reference (PDR) for Nonprescription Drugs and Dietary Supplements*. Montvale, NJ: Thomson.

Ulene, A. (2000). *Complete Guide to Vitamins, Minerals, and Herbs*. New York: Avery Books.

Weil, A. (2007). *8 Weeks to Optimum Health: A Proven Program of Taking Full Advantage of Your Body's Natural Healing Power*. New York: Alfred A. Knopf Publishers.

Resources

American Council on Science and Health
1995 Broadway
New York, NY 10023
212-362-7044
www.acsh.org

This covers many issues regarding nutrition and health with links to other sites.

Ask Dr. Weil Bulletin
www.drweil.com

The online information features Dr. Andrew Weil, founder of the Integrative Medicine Program, University of Arizona Health Sciences Center, Tucson, AZ. Offers many topics on integrative medicine and health.

National Heart, Lung, and Blood Institute
P.O. Box 30105
Bethesda, MD 20824-0105
301-592-8573
Facts About the DASH Eating Plan
www.nhlbi.nih.gov

This site offers the DASH diet plan with recipe suggestions for downloading or to order by mail.

Healthfinder Web Page
www.healthfinder.gov

Online consumer health information service provided by U.S. Department of Health and Human Services. Links to medical journals and databases with special resources on health.

National Institutes of Health
Office of Dietary Supplements
9000 Rockville Pike
Bethesda, Maryland 20892
www.ods.od.nih.gov

The International Bibliographic Information on Dietary Supplements database provides access to bibliographic citations and abstracts from published international, scientific literature on dietary supplements. This database was set up to help consumers, healthcare providers, educators, and researchers.

National Library of Medicine
8600 Rockville Pike
Bethesda, MD 20894
www.nlm.nih.gov

Nutrient Data Laboratory USDA Agricultural Research Service, Beltsville Human Nutrition Research Center
4700 River Rd., Unit 89
Riverdale, MD 20737
301-734-8491
www.nal.usda.gov/fnic/foodcomp/

This database gives facts about the composition of food, a glossary of terms, and links to other agencies.

PlaneTree Health Library
Mission Oaks
15891 Los Gatos-Almaden Rd.
Los Gatos, CA 95032
408-358-5667
www.planetreesanjose.org

This is a consumer health and medical library that is free and open to the public with the aim of providing access to information to make informed decisions about health. There is a range of information from professional/technical to easy-to-understand materials for all areas of medical treatment. They also offer some materials in Spanish and Vietnamese.

Chapter 4

Exercise: Mindfulness in Movement

OBJECTIVES

This chapter should enable you to

· List at least 10 benefits of regular physical activity

· Describe rib cage breathing

· Define aerobic exercise

· Calculate target heart rate

· List at least six activities that provide an aerobic workout

· State an example of a muscle-strengthening exercise

· Describe the benefits of Hatha Yoga and T'ai Chi Chuan

The body is designed to move. As you read this page, your heart is pumping. Blood is coursing through hundreds of miles of the cardiovascular network. Your lungs are expanding and contracting. Your eyes are moving. Your eardrums are vibrating, and neurons are firing. Thousands of processes are transpiring to promote the essence of your being . . . and you have not even lifted a finger to turn a page.

The body is not intended to be stagnant. Every movement, each effort of the muscles to pump blood brings the life force to every cell and flushes or removes from the body all that is no longer needed.

What does it mean to exercise? How does it change us? Why does the body require exercise? What does it look and feel like? These are questions to explore when using a model for holistic movement that is life-sustaining and promotes wellness.

REFLECTION

What attitude do you have toward exercise? What about your family background, experiences, and education contributed to that attitude?

What Does It Mean to Exercise?

For the last several decades, the public has been bombarded with the importance of exercise. In the 1960s, President John F. Kennedy implemented the President's Council on Physical Fitness, which launched the fitness craze. Children were tested and rewarded for their ability to climb a rope, do sit-ups and push-ups, throw a softball, and speedily run the 100-yard dash. This was the country's attempt to address the health hazards of a sedentary lifestyle for children. Today, physical fitness of youth remains an unmet goal. The United States has an increasingly overweight population with evidence of hypertension and atherosclerosis beginning in the childhood years. Lifestyle-related diseases are beginning earlier as people become increasingly physically inactive and technologically dependent. Labor-saving devices are not life-saving, and significant physical and spiritual deterioration is evident among all ages.

Improved physical fitness also has been a priority for those interested in positively impacting the aging process. Congress, in 1975, broadened the definition of the Older Americans Act to include ". . . services designed to enable older persons to attain and maintain physical and mental well being through programs of regular physical activity and exercise." In this new millennium, it is now more evident than ever that the country must reconsider its commitment to a healthy population for all citizens: young, old, rich, poor, and all ethnic populations that make up the diverse tapestry of the United States.

KEY POINT

Research shows that benefits of regular physical activity include improved cardiopulmonary function, reduced risk of coronary artery disease, lowered risk of colon cancer, heightened immune function, decreased susceptibility to depression, increased self-esteem, and improved quality of life.

Fitness is not limited to youth; growing old is not synonymous with a loss of good physical condition and function. Furthermore, it is a misconception that persons with physical limitations cannot engage in a health-promoting movement activity. Aging or disease does not mean weakening or sacrificing the abundance life has to offer. Hypertension control, bone and muscle strength, recovery from illness and injury, weight management, functional ability, and a general sense of well-being are all enhanced with regular physical activity.

Gentle movement programs can produce an enhanced immune response that is vital for resilience and physical/emotional integrity. Muscles respond to movement—the demand to contract and relax. Muscles are made to work, and just as the human spirit thrives when given a task or job to do, so does the body when put into motion.

> **KEY POINT**
>
> It is a myth that an aging person must experience physical decline, dysfunction, disability, and dependency. These outcomes are related to inactivity and a sedentary lifestyle—not the person's chronological age.

Commonly held, although limited, definitions of exercise bring images of calisthenics, sweaty workouts to loud music, strenuous weight lifting, and sessions of breathlessness to near exhaustion. It is time to evolve into a new view of exercise that is gentler and deeper and lasts a lifetime. This revised view emphasizes the significance of movement that engages the muscles and enhances the flow of body fluids and energy. Insufficient movement can show its effects in all areas of the self. Immobility causes muscles to shorten and weaken and joints to become stiff and less able to move or rotate smoothly. Sluggish digestion, slower elimination, and removal of toxins and waste products are outgrowths of inactivity. Inadequate physical movement affects the mind as well—evidenced by mild depression or a lack of enthusiasm and zest for living.

> **KEY POINT**
>
> *To keep the body in good health is a duty. . . . Otherwise we shall not be able to keep our minds strong and clear.*
>
> —*BUDDHA*

Benefits of Exercise

There are many benefits to exercise. Regular physical activity improves muscle strength and tone. Regular deliberate movement tones muscles, which has a positive impact on appearance, posture, body image, and the ability to engage in self-care activities. Exercise improves the efficiency of the body's metabolism. It helps use fat for fuel, and when you eat nutritious meals, it uses the energy for activity.

Regular aerobic exercise helps to regulate blood sugar or glucose levels. The increased demand for oxygen during exercise (which is what makes movement aerobic) improves the regulation and use of insulin, necessities for bringing glucose into the cells for metabolism or energy production. Exercise helps stabilize and keep the body's blood sugar levels balanced. Developing a regular movement program is a major preventative measure for adult-onset diabetes, heart disease, and atherosclerosis, as well as disorders of mood and thinking.

Endurance is enhanced by regular aerobic exercise. Exercise helps increase the efficiency of the heart and lungs, aiding in creating a greater capacity for coping with life challenges.

KEY POINT

When regularly challenged through aerobic activity (jumping, walking, jogging, biking, swimming, etc.), the heart and lungs learn to accommodate the body's increased demand for oxygen.

Oxygen is the essence of the life force; every cell of the body requires it for proper functioning. The gentle exertion of exercise challenges the organs to work more efficiently to draw the oxygen in more rapidly. Heart rate, breathing rate, and circulation increase, thereby allowing each cell to receive nourishment and eliminate wastes.

There is also a dilation or widening effect to the blood vessels because the heightened demand for oxygen causes the vessels to open wider to accommodate the increased fluid flow. Openness promotes flow. Again, let metaphor bring wisdom and empowerment to a holistic lifestyle. When the mind/body is open, it can receive new information and new possibilities, more of what is necessary and good. Strength and endurance become characteristics for the whole person, not just of the physical being, but also of emotional and spiritual facets.

Blood and lymphatic fluids carry the oxygen and nutrients necessary for the feeding of every cell. These fluids are the vehicles for the removal of all unnecessary and unwanted waste products from the body. The increased demand for blood flow stimulates the bone marrow to produce more blood cells to carry the oxygen. In a very short period of time, usually less than one month, improvements in cardiopulmonary function can be experienced. This challenge to the heart and lungs makes them stronger and more efficient. At rest, their rate goes down, meaning that they need to work less to get the same amount of work done. For this reason, resting blood pressure decreases. Weight-bearing/resistance activities, such as walking, swimming, weight training, jumping, running, yoga, and T'ai Chi, enhance the ability of the bones to keep calcium in the skeleton. A regular movement program is a major factor in the prevention of osteoporosis.

Exercise stimulates the circulation of endorphins—the neurohormonal transmitters responsible for feelings of well-being and psychospiritual hardiness, which can relieve stress. (For more information on stress, see Chapter 6: Flowing with the Reality of Stress.)

Regular exercise helps reduce chronic physical pain. Premenstrual cramping, headache, and joint stiffness can be relieved by movement. It can also help to prevent falls or injuries and shorten recovery time. The fit body is more resilient to the effects of gravity. Having the strength and balance to recover from falls is an important advantage to being in good physical condition.

Social, psychological, and emotional benefits are derived from exercise. The release of hormones and various neuropeptides from regular activity help decrease pain, alleviate anxiety, promote feelings of well-being, and suppress fatigue. Exercise improves circulation to the brain, which enhances alertness, clarity of thought, and memory; it sharpens the mind. It increases "regularity" and "flow" of the gastrointestinal tract, which assists with digestion and bowel elimination.

Exercise promotes the flow of lymph fluid. Lymph fluid is not driven by a pump like the heart, rather it undulates, or moves in wave-like fashion, in response to muscle contraction. The lymph pathways are laced within the body much like a fishnet stocking from the top of the head to the bottom of the toes. Lymph fluid flows from deep within to the superficial layers of the skin and returns back to the thoracic duct in the neck. From the thoracic duct, it joins with the general circulation. Circulation of fluid lubricates the joints, moistens the body—keeps us flowing within.

Exercise normalizes hormonal balance of the body. Not only is insulin better used for blood sugar stability, but cortisol, from the adrenal glands, is better modulated through aerobic activity. The modulation of cortisol is extremely important for reduction of the detrimental effects of stress. (Modulating cortisol is one of the important ways of keeping calcium in the bones and out of the blood stream where it tends to make the vascular system hard [atherosclerosis].)

What Does Exercise Look and Feel Like?

You do not need to sweat, pant, or hurt to benefit from action that is taken deliberately and in a context of wellness promotion. You simply need to develop a movement program that circulates fluid, contracts muscles, resists gravity, and symbolizes fun and value for you. This idea transcends the notion that exercise is done to give us the outside appearance of a "perfect body." The commercial world promotes an ideal body that is an unrealistic image for most people.

Movement is one of the nonnegotiable laws of life. The body, like all life forms, thrives on movement. It is a metaphor of life itself. There is an automatic rhythm within and outside us that does not cease until death—the cyclic motion of breathing, the expanding and contracting of lungs. It is only through the breath that we have life, and the more breath we have, the more vital and alive we feel.

REFLECTION

Take a moment right now, put down the book, let yourself get comfortable in your seat, and take a long deliberate inhalation in through your nose down to your lungs. Let your lungs be so full that you feel the entire rib cage rise and fill to capacity. Slowly let the air leave escape, and let your body sink in the exhalation. What do you observe about the effects?

The Mechanics of Breathing

The mechanics of breathing primarily involve the diaphragm—a large, dome-shaped muscle that separates the abdominal and chest cavities—and the intercostals, which are the muscles between the ribs. The process of inhaling and exhaling depends on the surface tension between the alveoli (air sacs of the lungs), the elasticity of the lungs within the chest wall, and the integrity of the large airways or bronchial tree to support the transport of air into the body.

When the diaphragm contracts or shortens, it flattens downward, increasing the chest cavity and creating a negative pressure that draws air into the lungs and produces the inspiration phase of the breathing cycle. Every breath inhaled can be considered an opportunity to "inspire the life force," to "bring in spirit" (inspiration) for the soul to be fed or nurtured through the energizing of the body (see Exhibit 4-1).

A conscious effort to deep breathe can be incorporated into activities, such as walking, yoga, T'ai Chi, dancing, swimming, jogging, or cycling. Diaphragmatic breathing is a potent health-promoting exercise and has benefits beyond helping to bring greater amounts of oxygen into the body.

There is a large collection of lymph nodes in the belly region. Each "full-bellied breath" massages this lymphatic center. The movement of the diaphragm "milks" the lymph fluid back up to the heart (see Chapter 5 for a discussion of the lymphatic system and the role of exercise in promoting healthy immune integrity).

Aerobic Exercise

Aerobic exercise is one of the most important and efficient methods of attaining muscular and cardiovascular fitness. Aerobic exercise is accomplished when enough demand is put on the muscles to increase their need for oxygen, causing the heart to beat faster and the lungs to work harder. This not only increases cardiovascular endurance, but also helps to

---

EXHIBIT 4-1 Rib Cage Breathing

Inhale deeply while raising your extended arms from your side to straight above your head. Exhale as your arms are returned to your side. Enjoy the sensation of a fully expanded rib cage. Keep the movement of the arms smooth and slow. Count 1 and 2 inhaling and moving the arms up; count 3 and 4 exhaling and moving the arms down. This is an excellent exercise for pulmonary hygiene—to expand the lungs fully, bringing oxygen to the very deepest aspects of the lungs. It is a wonderful way to cleanse lung tissue, bringing in life-giving oxygen and flushing out waste products that no longer serve the body. Do rib cage breathing four to six times to a session. It is a powerful way to renew and refresh as well as to put the lungs and ribs through their "full range of function."

prevent heart attacks by strengthening the heart and increasing the flow of blood through the vascular system, thereby keeping the arteries open and elastic. Fresh oxygen in the blood improves the functioning of all cells in the body. It helps to burn away fat from the muscles and to build new, lean muscle tissue. This increases the metabolic rate of the entire body even during sleep and is valuable for losing weight and keeping it off.

In order to gain aerobic benefits, the heart rate must be elevated and maintained for the duration of the workout within the target heart rate. The target heart rate range is the range between the maximum and minimum calculated heart rate based on age. When an aerobic exercise is started, a person should keep the heart rate down toward the lower end of the range, gradually moving toward the higher.

KEY POINT

To find your target heart rate, subtract your age from 220. This gives you your maximum heart rate. Multiply your maximum heart rate by 0.50 and 0.75 to get your target heart rate range.

To get aerobic, it is easiest to use the legs; because the quadriceps are the largest muscles of the body, they require the most oxygen and thus will burn the greatest amount of energy in the shortest amount of time. Examples of moderate activities that use the legs and provide an aerobic workout are listed in Exhibit 4-2.

Rebounding or jumping on a trampoline is a particularly beneficial form of exercise. Most forms of aerobic exercise demand the body move forward, or horizontally, along the earth. Running, cycling, swimming, or walking allows the body to move in a measurable distance. Jumping on a rebounder or trampoline, on the other hand, gives the body the

---

EXHIBIT 4-2   Activities for Aerobic Exercise

- Fast dancing for 30 minutes
- Swimming laps for 20 minutes; water aerobics for 30 minutes
- Walking—this includes on a treadmill—for 2 miles in 30 minutes
- Bicycling—either outside or on a stationary bike—for 5 miles in 30 minutes
- Stair walking for 15 minutes
- Jumping rope or jumping on a trampoline for 15 minutes
- Ball sports, such as tennis, handball, racquetball, soccer, or basketball for 15 minutes
- Jogging or running 1.5 miles in 15 minutes

unique experience of moving vertically, allowing gravity to act on the cells, tissues, organs, and muscles in a way that literally squeezes out toxins and waste products. This activity also challenges every cell in the body (approximately 60 trillion) to improve integrity, strength, and function. The action of jumping up and down causes the body to adapt to and resist the force of gravity. This act of resistance promotes stronger bones, firmer muscles, and improvement in the circulation of all body fluids. Jumping or rebounding puts exceptional challenge on the venous and lymphatic systems to return the blood and lymph back to the heart. The main restriction to someone developing a rebounding program is lower back pain or injury. Lumbar back injury or strain would prohibit safe and enjoyable jumping.

By engaging in a moderate aerobic activity for at least 20 to 30 minutes a day for 3 to 5 days a week, improvements in all areas of mind/body/spirit will be noticed. Changes can usually be seen after three to five weeks of starting the exercise program.

KEY POINT

Any aerobic activity you choose will serve you well if you enjoy doing it. There is no "right or wrong" movement, if you pay attention to your body. Pain, injury, and discontent are the symptoms of an inappropriate activity. Joy, enthusiasm, and commitment to the habit are indications that an aerobic activity is a well-suited one.

Muscle Strengthening Exercises

Strength is an essential, functional component of much of what we do. The lack of strength is responsible for many injuries. Weight training is useful in developing muscle strength. Lifting weights is good for increasing the size and strength of specific muscles. This kind of training can be useful for people who wish to develop particular muscles or muscle groups for a specific sport in which they are involved. It also is used for bodybuilding.

KEY POINT

· Muscle bulk is attained by using weights, doing 12 to 20 repetitions.
· Muscle strength is developed by using the heaviest weights manageable by the person, doing 2 to 6 repetitions.
· Muscle endurance and definition is increased by lighter weights, while doing 40–50 repetitions.

When working out, the principle of overload must be employed. That is, the number of repetitions, the amount of weight, and the speed and intensity of the effort must continually increase if there is to be any real benefit from the practice.

Energy-Building Exercises

Exercise systems such as Hatha yoga and T'ai Chi Chuan are aimed at the development of energy that flows through the external body structure. The process of Qi (or Chi) development produces an effect in the physical body often seen as increased strength, attention, endurance, and vitality. As you work on your energy, you will enhance your physical body.

Hatha yoga develops poise, balance, strength, and amazing agility and limberness. The postures (asanas) massage and revitalize the internal organs and harmonize the Qi of the body, imparting internal strength and youthfulness. There is no strain as one assumes the postures and lets the muscles relax and stretch into place. Special attention is paid to alignment of the spine and development of spinal flexibility because the spine is the center of the energetic and nervous systems and energy blocked here affects the entire system.

Through T'ai Chi Chuan, some of the world's most advanced techniques for the training of the mind and body in harmony are available. In Taoist philosophy, the T'ai Chi, or the source and terminus of the universe manifest as a unity, is composed of two interacting and complementary forces called yin and yang. In T'ai Chi Chuan, this idea is expressed through a beautiful, coordinated series of postures that through regular practice develop and coordinate the body, under the control of Qi, to a level of perfection not otherwise attainable. Proper alignment of the spine is maintained, and the mind is stilled through the slowness of movement with the focus of attention placed on the lower abdomen.

Any Activity Can Benefit Your Health

Regular structured activity, such as walking, yoga, swimming, trampoline jumping, T'ai Chi, or any number of other movement programs enhances health by causing

- Muscles to grow
- Metabolism to increase, causing more efficient use of the energy of food
- Fat stores to be reduced
- Blood vessels to multiply
- Bones to stay harder
- Thinking processes to be sharper
- Mood to be positive and elevated

An exercise program also promotes vitality and enthusiasm in your relationships. Just as movement of fluids flushes toxins out and allows energy to flow more freely into you, it also opens your social experiences by increasing your confidence and sense of competence.

KEY POINT

The yin/yang concept of balance is promoted in many Eastern philosophies. Applying some of these concepts to movement is helpful when developing a lifestyle fitness program.

Yang energy is assertive, thrusts outward, is masculine in nature, and is supportive. It is strength and protection—the ability to "stand up for oneself." Developing an aerobic exercise program that uses the largest muscles of the body (thighs or quadriceps) most efficiently circulates blood, strengthens the cardiovasculature, releases toxins through sweat, and in general promotes strength, endurance, and resilience. It is yang activity.

Yin activity, the softer type, is just as necessary for a balanced life. Examples include T'ai Chi and other forms of "moving meditation" and yoga. Yin activity brings oneself inward and quiet. It develops focus, balance, and a sense of "center."

Lifetime fitness means to be active throughout the life span. All that is needed for a lifetime fitness program is finding the activity that resonates with the heart's desire to move. It is best to do the chosen activity at least three to four times a week, month to month, season to season. It does not take long for the activity to become a habit. Maintaining a regular, realistic, and pleasurable movement program is a key to radiant health. Each individual is the best care provider and custodian of his or her own heart and soul.

Summary

Physical fitness is important for people of all ages. Exercise strengthens and tones muscles, improves efficiency of body, enhances cardiovascular function, prevents bone loss, relieves stress, helps reduce chronic pain, speeds healing, elevates mood, sharpens the mind, increases regularity and flow of the gastrointestinal system, promotes lymphatic fluid flow, and normalizes the body's hormonal balance.

Aerobic exercise involves putting ample demand on the muscles to increase their oxygen requirement, thereby causing the heart and lungs to work harder. To gain benefit from aerobic exercise, the heart rate should be maintained within the target heart rate range during exercise. Target heart rate range is the range between maximum and minimum heart rate, calculated by using the individual's age. Other forms of exercise include weight training, which is useful in developing muscle strength, and Hatha yoga and T'ai Chi Chuan, to enhance energy flow. Exercise plans that are sustainable and most effective are those that are regular, realistic, pleasurable, and individualized.

Suggested Reading

Anderson, B., Anderson, J., & Turlington, C. (2003). *Stretching.* Bolinas, CA: Shelter Publications.

Brooks, L. (1999). *Rebounding to Better Health.* Albuquerque, NM: Ke Publishers.

Chia, M. (2005). *The Inner Structure of Tai Chi: Mastering the Classic Forms of Tai Chi Chi Kung.* Huntington, NY: Healing Tao Books.

Hahn, F., Eades, M. R., & Eades, M. D. (2002). *The Slow Burn Fitness Revolution: The Slow Motion Exercise That Will Change Your Body in 30 Minutes a Week.* New York: Broadway Books.

Isacowitz, R. (2006). *Pilates.* Champaign, IL: Human Kinetics.

Jahnke, R. (2002). *The Healing Promise of Qi: Creating Extraordinary Wellness Through Tai Chi and Qigong.* New York: McGraw-Hill Contemporary Books.

Khalsa, S. K. (2000). *Kundalini Yoga.* Darya Ganj, New Delhi: DK Publishers.

Kisner, C., & Colby, L.A. (2007). *Therapeutic Exercise: Foundations and Techniques.* Philadelphia: F.A. Davis.

Kirsh, D. (2004). *Sound Mind, Sound Body: David Kirsh's Ultimate 6-Week Fitness Transformation for Men and Women.* New York: Rodale Press.

Siler, B. (2000). *The Pilates Body: The Ultimate At-Home Guide to Strengthening, Lengthening, and Toning Your Body without Machines.* New York: Doubleday.

Simon, H. (2007). *The No Sweat Exercise Plan: Harvard Medical School Guides.* New York: McGraw-Hill.

Chapter 5

Immune Enhancement: Mind/Body Considerations

OBJECTIVES

This chapter should enable you to

· Describe the peripheral lymphatic system

· Describe diaphragmatic breathing

· List at least three signs of an imbalanced immune system

The germ is nothing. . . . The terrain is everything.

LOUIS PASTEUR

It is your immune system's resilience that protects you from overwhelming infections that can knock you out cold in the ring of life's daily matches. Your susceptibility to infections and diseases, from the simple cold to catastrophic cancers, is deeply influenced by the health and integrity of the immune system. Likewise, chronic diseases and imbalances can threaten the immune system.

The reflective saying "as within—so without" represents a way of understanding immune function. Immune integrity can be viewed as a metaphor of your ability to "stand up for yourself." Just as you need to have a good communication network in your personal and professional lives, you also need exquisite communication pathways between each cell and system within the body.

The immune system represents an understanding of "boundaries" and harmonious living in community with others. Your integrity, resilience, and support lie within the immune system's ability to mobilize, defend, communicate, and hold peace and balance within. A primary role of the immune system is to "serve and protect." The capacity and success of this system to function optimally and be ever vigilant are important aspects of radiant health.

Components of the Immune System

The immune system consists of a lacy network of pathways capable of transporting immune cells throughout the body. It also has a collection of organs, tissues, and cells dispersed strategically throughout the body (see Table 5-1). This system is intricately connected to the nervous system (brain) and the endocrine system (hormonal).

The lymph fluid of the body is constantly "oozing" toward the heart from the farthest reaches of the body and is then reintroduced into the general lymphatic circulation. Two layers of lacy lymph networks are just under the skin, and these return the lymph fluid to

TABLE 5-1 The Immune System

Component	Function
Spleen	Bloody organ in the upper left quadrant of the abdomen that produces antibodies, maintains cellular immunity, recirculates white blood cells, and receives B cells, T cells, antigens, macrophages, and antigen-reactive cells from the blood.
Bone marrow	Located in the hollow interior of the long bones, produces red blood cells and macrophages; B and T cells undergo development here.
Lymph nodes	Pea-shaped organs throughout the body that are connected by a network of vessels that receive drainage and filter antigens from this lymphatic fluid.
Thymus gland	Located beneath the breastbone, this gland reaches its full size in early childhood and then progressively shrinks. It produces and stores T cells.
Other organs	Tonsils are groups of lymphoid tissues located in the throat that contain B and T cells. The appendix, Peyer's patches (accumulations of lymphoid cells under mucous membranes that produce nodules), and intestinal nodes are sites of B-cell maturation and antibody production for the intestinal region.
Cells	
Macrophages	Large white blood cells produced in bone marrow, responsible for phagocytosis.
B cells	Bone marrow–derived cells that produce antibodies that neutralize or destroy antigens.
T cells	Thymus-derived cells consist of T-helper cells that induce B cells to respond to an antigen and T-suppressor cells that halt specific activity of immunologic response. T-helper and T-suppressor cells are in a delicate balance that must be maintained for adequate immune response.
NK (natural killer) cells	NK cells kill foreign invaders on direct contact without B cell involvement by producing cytotoxin, a cell poison.

the heart. The purpose of these redundant lymphatic pathways is to provide a passage for the return of lymph fluid to the heart.

Keep in mind that lymph fluid is the consistency of an egg white—it is quite thick and moves very slowly. Lymphatic fluid does not have a pump to force it through the body like the heart forces blood with every beat. Lymph fluid movement is dependent on the muscles that provide movement.

Function of the Lymphatic System

All lymph fluid passes through lymph nodes. The lymph nodes are depots where special white blood cells, called T cells, wait on alert for foreign material, such as bacteria or viruses, to be brought into the nodes for identification and security check.

Lymph nodes are located strategically throughout the body. Seventy percent of the body's immune system surrounds the abdominal area. A large number of lymph nodes and vessels are in the gut to make sure that all the foreign, non-self material that is ingested becomes user friendly and beneficial. Imagine the amount of infection and disease that you could suffer if you did not have strong, vigilant immunity to counter all of the bacteria and other foreign material that is carried on food or produced by the process of digestion.

The rest of the body's lymph nodes are located where major bones articulate, or meet, and where the body has openings to the outside world. Lymph nodes are at the ankles, knees, around the groin area, elbows, armpits, and chest, and chains of lymph nodes are along the neck and collarbone.

There are two reasons lymph fluid must pass through nodes on its return trip to the heart. One is to carry protein molecules to the general circulation because proteins are too big to be circulated back through the venous circulation. This helps keep the fluid levels of the body balanced. The second reason that all lymph fluid passes through lymph nodes is to identify pathogens (bacteria, fungi, viruses) that are foreign to the body.

The purpose of immune cells is to recognize what is self and what is not self. Just as the eyes sense or recognize what is outside of self and retain a memory of that image for life, so, too, the immune cells recognize and remember for a lifetime an encounter with a particular organism—whether be it a bacteria, virus, fungi, food, or an environmental allergen. Your immunity provides you with the surveillance mechanism to defend and protect from the day you are born until your last breath.

The immune system is intimately connected to the nervous and endocrine systems. Not only does it respond to physical factors, such as invading pathogens or germs, but also it is very sensitive to your thoughts and emotions. How you think and decide to interpret the world around you influences the kind of activity that either enhances immune resilience or promotes immune disorders.

The immune cells are on patrol and in action every day of your life. They do not die off like skin cells, organ cells, and most other cells of the body that have a particular life span ranging from a day to a few months. Immune cells always perceive and remember the biochemical interactions between self and substances foreign to the body. The cells are mobile and, when optimal conditions exist, able to transport unwanted materials from the body, keeping the host victorious against infection or compromise.

KEY POINT

It is the job of the immune system to protect the body from disease.

Enhancing Lymphatic Flow

The most important muscle for the movement of your immune system is the diaphragm—the thin, dome-shaped muscle that separates the lungs from the abdominal cavity like a parachute. Every deep breath and every step that you take has the effect of massaging or oozing lymph fluid along its way. Vigorous deep breathing, as occurs during brisk walking or any aerobic activity, or conscious breathing, such as that done in yoga and other meditative practices, enhances the flow of lymph fluid through a type of breathing called diaphragmatic or belly breathing. Babies come into the world belly breathing, and it is something that needs to be relearned to promote optimal immune function. Deep breathing with the diaphragm is an activity that is extremely useful in improving immune integrity.

KEY POINT

Diaphragmatic breathing is the process of contracting the diaphragm, the thin, dome-shaped muscle covering the stomach and liver, to create a deep inhalation. During the in breath, an effort is made to push the stomach out as the diaphragm flattens down onto the abdomen. This enables the lungs to expand more fully. The rhythm produced by this breathing enhances lymphatic fluid movement and helps milk the removal of toxins and waste products from lymph fluid.

Making a habit of practicing belly breathing is a powerful yet subtle means of stress management. Deep breathing helps the heart beat more regularly and perform more competently. Carbon dioxide is more efficiently removed with diaphragmatic breathing. One will be more alert and fit when the breath is attuned with other rhythms of the body. Changing the breathing style to belly breathing rather than chest breathing will bring more oxygen into the cells, increase the energy available for activity and performance, and enhance the innate harmony between breath, heart rate, sense of well-being, and enthusiasm for life. Belly breathing promotes relaxation and maintains calmness in situations of perceived stress through the action of the diaphragm synchronizing its rhythm with the heart's rhythm and other processes of the body. A state of peace and harmony helps to conserve the immune system.

Physical exercise has the ability to increase the vessels that carry blood and lymph fluid throughout the body. The more vessels available to carry blood and lymph fluid, the more efficiently the heart functions and fluids flow. Just as the Dan Ryan Expressway in Chicago opens its collaterals or extra lanes to accommodate the increased number of vehicles, the body also has the ability to develop collateral circulation to relieve congestion and keep the flow moving easily and effortlessly.

KEY POINT

The job of the peripheral lymphatic system is to clear germs and cancer cells from the body. This lacy network accomplishes this through the massaging movement of the muscles of motion and breathing. Regular physical activity and deep breathing help the efforts of the immune system.

Signs of Imbalanced Immune Function

You may be beginning to notice a relationship between immune integrity, exercise, nutrition, positive attitude, and the other aspects of healthful living. The body and mind are an interconnecting network of systems affecting each other and making up the total being. It is the immune system's lacy network covering the body from the top of the head to the tips of the toes that links the nervous and endocrine systems with thoughts and perceptions. This is why consideration of how well people are in rhythm with themselves and life around them is of equal importance as the quality of the air they breathe or the amount of exercise they get. Social alienation is compromising to the immune system. For example, it has been shown that spouses have a much greater chance of becoming gravely ill during the first year after the loss of their mate than other persons in the same age group. Loneliness and the lack of feeling that you belong to others is as depleting of the immune system as any other essential nutrient deficiency.

REFLECTION

Immune integrity has as much to do with the quality of your relationships as it does with the quality of your air and water. Are you as concerned about your psychosocial environment as you are with your physical environment?

Exhibit 5-1 Questions to Reveal Imbalances of Mind and Spirit

· **Disorientation.** Are you feeling disconnected to your life's calling, your life's purpose? Do you love the work you do or do you grudgingly face the world each day with a dark feeling of being out of sync? Is energy flowing abundantly through you or steadily being drained without replenishment?

· **Disorganization.** Look around you. Does your house and office reflect how you feel about your home or your work? Are your living and work spaces organized and manageable, or are you overwhelmed and taken over by stuff that no longer serves you? Do your possessions create a sense of peace and sacredness or bring you stress and frustration?

· **Disidentification.** Are you working on becoming the person you truly want to be? Are you honoring your life's calling? Are you tending to all the others in your life and ignoring your own needs? Do you nourish your spirit and soul?

· **Disintegration.** Are you feeling more torn down than renewed? Do you have regular infections? Are you chronically tired or fatigued? Is there an air of zest and enthusiasm in your daily life?

In addition to physical signs of disease, there are symptoms affecting the mind and spirit that can help people to realize that they are not in balance; these can be categorized under the headings of *disorientation*, *disorganization*, *disidentification*, and *disintegration*. Some questions that can aid in exploring the presence of imbalance are described in Exhibit 5-1.

Boosting Immunologic Health

Diet

In addition to a good basic diet, some foods can positively affect immunity. These include milk, yogurt, nonfat cottage cheese, eggs, fresh fruits and vegetables, nuts, garlic, onions, sprouts, pure honey, and unsulfured molasses. A daily multivitamin and mineral supplement is also helpful; specific nutrients that have immune-boosting effects are listed in Exhibit 5-2. Because of their negative effect on the immune system, the intake of refined carbohydrates, saturated and polyunsaturated fats, caffeine, and alcohol should be limited.

Fasting

Fasting, the abstinence of solid foods for one to two days, is becoming increasingly popular as a means to promote health and healing. The effects of fasting on the immune system include the following:

- Increased macrophage activity and neutrophil antibacterial activity
- Raised immunoglobulin levels
- Improvement of cell-mediated immunity, ability of monocytes to kill bacteria, and natural killer cell activity
- Reductions in free radicals and antioxidant damage

For most persons, a day or two without food is safe; however, an assessment of health status is essential before beginning a fast because some health conditions and medication needs can be altered. Also, it is essential that good fluid intake be maintained during a fast.

Exercise

Any form of exercise, done regularly, can be of benefit to the immune system. Exercise need not be strenuous; low-impact exercise, such as yoga and T'ai Chi, has a positive effect on immunity (see Chapter 4 for more information about exercise).

Stress Management

The thymus, spleen, and lymph nodes are involved in the stress response; therefore, stress can affect the function of the immune system. Some stress-related diseases, including arthritis, depression, hypertension, and diabetes mellitus, cause a rise in serum cortisol, a powerful immunosuppressant. Elevated cortisol levels can lead to a breakdown in lymphoid tissue, inhibition of the production of natural killer cells, increases in T-suppressor cells, and reductions in the levels of T-helper cells and virus-fighting interferon.

Individuals need to identify stress reduction measures with which they are comfortable so that they will practice them on a regular basis. It makes no sense for a person to attempt to engage in meditation if he or she is uncomfortable with that activity because it will be

---

EXHIBIT 5-2   Immune-Enhancing Nutrients

Protein
Vitamins A, E, B_1, B_2, B_6, B_{12}, C
Folic acid
Pantothenic acid
Iron
Magnesium
Manganese
Selenium
Zinc

more stress producing than stress reducing. Some stress-reduction measures that could be used are progressive relaxation, meditation, prayer, yoga, imagery, exercise, diversional activity, and substitution of caffeine and junk foods with juices and nutritious snacks.

KEY POINT

The ability of our psychological state to affect physical health is recognized; in fact, the specialty of psychoneuroimmunology has emerged in recognition of the fact that thoughts and emotions affect the immune system.

Psychological Traits and Predispositions

Studies have identified traits consistent with strong immune systems to include the following[1,2]:

- Assertiveness
- Faith in God or a higher power
- Ability to trust and offer unconditional love
- Willingness to be open and confide in others
- Purposeful activity
- Control over one's life
- Acceptance of stress as a challenge rather than a threat
- Altruism
- Development and exercise of multiple facets of personality

Individuals could improve their immune health by developing and nurturing some of these characteristics.

REFLECTION

How many traits consistent with a strong immune system do you possess? What can you do to nurture those traits and to develop additional ones?

Caring for the Immune System by Caring for Self

As people support and nurture themselves, their immune systems will respond by helping them to feel:

- **Reorientated:** A renewed sense of belonging and purpose. Perceptions of belonging and connectiveness help people feel grounded and secure. This is in contrast to having perceptions of alienation and aloneness, which cause the immune system to stay vigilant and on the defense, which can be an exhausting stance over time.

- **Reorganized:** Being able to discern what is and is not truly needed for one's highest good. This can include letting go of what no longer serves one whether it is old clothes, appliances, or relationships that tear down instead of building up and making revisions on priorities in life. These are ways that people can empower themselves without the stress of trying to take charge over those things that cannot be controlled.

- **Reidentified:** A renewed definition of one's identity and purpose. This can be achieved through developing ways of nourishing your body, mind, and spirit. Meditation, solitude, and prayer are among the practices that can assist with this.

- **Reintegrated:** A renewed belief and confidence in self. As the mind/body is supplied with what it needs for optimal function, there is renewal of hope and zest for life. Reducing the fear and anxiety that people feel about daily life eases the burden on the immune system by reducing its need to protect and defend.

It is the ability to adapt and endure that gives people healing powers to recover from disease and move from darkness into light. Beliefs can lay the foundation for the body to restructure or reform its physical self. How people think and feel connected has an enormous influence on the strength and vitality of immune function. The health and well-being of the mind and spirit can be just as important to the immune response as nutrition or immune-boosting herbs such as echinacea.

A variety of additional measures can assist in enhancing the function of the immune system. Some of these are discussed in the chapters about healthful nutrition (see Chapter 2), exercise (see Chapter 4), flowing with the reality of stress (see Chapter 6), herbal remedies (see Chapter 22), and environmental effects on the immune system (see Chapter 12).

Summary

The immune system is a lacy network consisting of organs, tissues, and cells. It monitors the body for disease-producing organisms and initiates defenses to eliminate them. It is helpful for people to be concerned about the health of their immune systems and to engage in practices to promote immune health. Physical exercise and diaphragmatic breathing promote the movement of lymphatic fluid throughout the body.

Individuals can take action to enhance their immune function, such as eating specific foods, fasting, exercising, managing stress, and developing psychological traits consistent with strong immunity.

An imbalanced immune system can create a variety of physical signs, such as increased ease and frequency of infection. In addition to physical signs, an imbalanced immune system can cause disorientation, disorganization, disidentification, and disintegration.

References

1. Cohen, S., & Miller, G. E. (2001). Stress, immunity, and susceptibility to upper respiratory infections. In Ader, R., Felten, D., & Cohen, N. (eds.), *Psychoneuroimmunology*, 3rd ed. NY: Academic Press.
2. Friedman, H. S. (2007). The multiple linkages of personality and disease. Brain, Behavior and Immunity. Retrieved October 18, 2007 from www.sciencedirect.com

Suggested Reading

Ader, R. (ed.). (2006). *Psychoneuroimmunology,* 4th ed. New York: Academic Press.

Alford, L. (2007). Findings of interest from immunology and psychoneuroimmunology. *Manual Therapy, 12*(2):176–180.

Avitsur, R., Padgett, D. A., & Sheridan, J. F. (2006). Social interactions, stress, and immunity. *Neurologic Clinics, 24*(3):483–491.

Cohen, N, (2006). Norman Cousins Lecture. The uses and abuses of psychoneuroimmunology: a global overview. *Brain, Behavior, and Immunity, 20*(2):99–112.

Cott, A. (2007). *Fasting: the Ultimate Diet.* Winter Park, FL: Hastings House.

Daruna, J. (2004). *Introduction to Psychoneurology.* Burlington, MA: Elsevier Academic Press.

Godbout, J. B., & Johnson, R. W. (2006). Age and neuroinflammation: a lifetime of psychoneuroimmune consequences. *Neurologic Clinics, 24*(3):521–538.

Gold, S. M., & Irwin, M. R. (2006). Depression and immunity: inflammation and depressive symptoms in multiple sclerosis. *Neurologic Clinics, 24*(3):507–519.

Goldsby, R. A., Marcus, D. A., Kindt, T. J., & Kuby, J. (2003). *Immunology.* New York: W.H. Freeman and Company.

Jason, E., and Ketcham, K. (1999). *Chinese Medicine for Maximum Immunity.* Three Rivers, MI: Three Rivers Press.

Langley, P. Fonseca, J., & Iphofen, R (2006). Psychoneuroimmunology and health from a nursing perspective. *British Journal of Nursing, 15*(20):1126–1129.

Moldawer, N., & Carr, E. (2000). The promise of recombinant interleukin-2. *American Journal of Nursing, 100*(5):35–40.

Novack, D. H., Cameron, O., Epel, E., Ader, R., Waldstein, S. R., Levenstein, S., Antoni, M. H., & Wainer, A. R. (2007). Psychosomatic medicine: the scientific foundation of the biopsychosocial model. *Academic Psychiatry, 31*(5):388–401.

Opp, M. R. (2006). Sleep and psychoneuroimmunology. *Neurologic Clinics, 24*(3):493–506.

Schniederman, N., Ironman, G., & Seigel, S. G. (2005). Stress and health: psychological, behavioral, and biological determinants. *Annual Review of Clinical Psychology, 1*:607–628.

Chapter 6

Flowing with the Reality of Stress

OBJECTIVES

This chapter should enable you to

· List the three stages of response to stress that D. Hans Selye identified
· Define *psychoneuroimmunology*
· Describe different types of stress
· Outline the response of the sympathetic nervous system to stress
· Describe factors to consider in the self-assessment of stress
· List four common elements of stress-reduction measures
· Describe a progressive muscular relaxation exercise
· List at least three measures that can aid in stress reduction

Stress is an inescapable reality of the average life. On a daily basis, people are exposed to numerous events, issues, and circumstances that challenge them. When faced with stress, some people seem to rise to the occasion and thrive, whereas others experience a myriad of negative physical and psychological effects. Why is this so? The answer, despite much research on the subject, is not clearly understood but is strongly connected to how an individual *manages* stress.

The Concept of Stress

In the 1950s, Dr. Hans Selye, recognized as the father of stress research, laid the foundation for much of the work that has since unfolded in the field of stress.[1] His premise was that all organisms have a similar response when confronted with a challenge to their well-being, regardless of whether that challenge was seen as positive or negative. He called that response the *general adaptation syndrome*, which he defined as "the manifestations of stress in the whole body, as they develop in time." He identified three stages of the general adaptation syndrome.

KEY POINT

The three stages of response to stress that Selye identified are the *alarm reaction*, the *stage of resistance*, and the *stage of exhaustion*.

The first stage is the *alarm reaction*, more commonly known as the fight-or-flight response, a physiologic process first described by a psychologist, Dr. Walter Cannon, in the early 1900s. In this stage, the body gears up physically and mentally for battle or energizes to escape the threat. Often referred to as an *adrenaline rush*, it can be recognized as the pounding heart, dry mouth, cold hands, and knot in the stomach felt when you perceive yourself to be threatened. In the *stage of resistance*, the body maintains a state of readiness, but not to the extent of the initial alarm reaction. If the threat is not eliminated and this heightened state of readiness persists, Selye believed that the *stage of exhaustion* would be reached. At this point, the body, having spent its existing energy reserves, is no longer able to sustain the workload of constant readiness. It is here that it may begin to fail, resulting in the onset of illness and possibly death.

Decades of continuing research into the mechanisms and effects of stress have yielded much information; however, interpretations of that information vary greatly and are sometimes considered controversial. A major development in the area is the field of *psychoneuroimmunology*—the study of the interaction between psychologic processes and the nervous and immune systems of the human body.[2] This has brought new definitions of stress that address the mind–body connection, such as one of the early ones offered by Seward that stress is "the inability to cope with a perceived or real (or imagined to be real) threat to one's mental, physical, emotional, or spiritual well-being, which results in a series of physiologic responses and adaptations."[3]

KEY POINT

Psychoneuroimmunology is the in-depth study of the interaction of the mind, the central nervous system, and the immune system, and their impact on our health and well-being.

Most authors and researchers now agree that there is a difference in the body's response to good stress and bad stress. Good stress (termed *eustress* by Selye) motivates and has pleasant or enjoyable effects, such as that resulting from a job promotion or a surprise birthday party. Although it causes an alarm response, the strength and duration of that response is usually short lived. Conversely, bad stress (termed *distress* by Selye), such as that experienced when involved in a confrontation with a spouse or being involved in a car accident, most often fully initiates the fight-or-flight response and may also have a prolonged impact on your well-being. This distress is what people usually are speaking of when they use the word *stress*.

Stress can also be viewed as *acute* or *chronic*. *Acute stress* has a sudden onset and is usually very intense but ends relatively quickly. The body quickly recovers, and the symptoms of acute stress subside. *Chronic stress* is stress that lasts over a prolonged period of time, but may not be as severe or intense as the acute type. Chronic stress is believed to be a major culprit in the development of stress-related diseases.[4]

> **KEY POINT**
>
> An example of acute stress could be losing your wallet containing your paycheck. Initially, when you discover you have lost your wallet, your stress level is very high. After you find your missing wallet under the front seat of your car, the crisis is over.
>
> A prolonged illness of a loved one or lengthy unemployment can cause chronic stress, exhausting all of your coping resources over time.

The Body's Physical Response to Stress

When your brain perceives a threat to your well-being, a series of events made up of chemical reactions and physical responses occurs rapidly. The first of these is the activation of your sympathetic nervous system, which stimulates the release of *epinephrine* from the outer layer of the adrenal gland (medulla) located on top of the kidney and *norepinephrine*, also from the adrenal glands and from the ends of nerves located throughout our bodies. When these hormones are released, the fight-or-flight response is triggered. Your heart, blood vessels, and lungs are strongly impacted by these hormones. The force and rate of the heart's contractions increase, and the rate and depth of our breathing increases. The *arteries*, vessels carrying oxygen and nutrient-rich blood to your vital organs, widen or dilate to ensure extra blood flow to the heart, lungs, and major muscles. At the same time, the arteries to areas that are not essential (the skin and digestive tract) narrow or constrict. This provides extra blood for the vital organs. One of the other major outcomes of sympathetic nervous system stimulation is a large increase in the production of glucose, your body's primary energy source. The overall net result is an increase in the available amount of glucose and oxygen for the organs and tissues that need it.

Additionally, the pituitary gland, located in the brain, is actively involved in the stress response. The anterior pituitary gland releases a hormone called *adrenocorticotrophic hormone*. This hormone stimulates the outer layer of the adrenal gland (cortex) to release *aldosterone* and *cortisol*. Aldosterone, along with a hormone produced by the posterior pituitary gland vasopressin or antidiuretic hormone, works to preserve blood volume by limiting the amount of salt and water the kidney is allowed to excrete. Cortisol increases the production of glucose and assists in the breakdown of fat and proteins to provide the additional energy needed to protect the body from the perceived threat. The hormones released during the stress response have many effects on the body (see Exhibit 6-1).

Sources of Stress

The sources of stress in daily life are different for each individual. One person may find a 20-mile drive home through a mountain pass after work tedious and frustrating, whereas

---

EXHIBIT 6-1   Effects of Stress

Physiologic

Increased heart rate, grinding of teeth, rise in blood pressure, insomnia, dryness of mouth and throat, anorexia, sweating, fatigue, tightness of chest, slumped posture, headache, pain, tightness in neck and back, nausea, vomiting, urinary frequency, indigestion, missed menstrual cycle, diarrhea, reduced interest in sex, trembling, twitching, and accident proneness

Emotional

Irritability, tendency to cry easily, depression, nightmares, angry outbursts, suspiciousness, emotional instability, jealousy, poor concentration, decreased social involvement, disinterest in activities, bickering, withdrawal, complaining, criticizing, restlessness, tendency to be easily startled, anxiety, increased smoking, increased use of sarcasm, and use of drugs or alcohol

Intellectual

Forgetfulness, errors in arithmetic and grammar, poor judgment, preoccupation, poor concentration, inattention to detail, reduced creativity, blocking, less fantasizing, reduced productivity

Work Habits

Increased lateness, absenteeism, low morale, depersonalization, avoidance of contact with coworkers, excess breaks, resistance to change, impatience, negative attitude, reluctance to assist others, carelessness, verbal or physical abuse, poor quality and quantity of work, threats to resign, resignation

Source: Eliopoulos, C. *Nursing Administration Manual for Long-Term Care Facilities*, 7th ed., Health Education Network, 2008. Reprinted with permission.

---

another may view it as a source of pleasure and relaxation. Other sources of stress can be associated with the physical environment, job, interpersonal relationships, past experiences, or psychological makeup. Identifying what stresses them and how they react to that stress is the first step for people to take in developing effective personal stress-management strategies. A variety of tools can help people to identify the stresses in their lives, one of which is offered in Exhibit 6-2.

REFLECTION

Take a few minutes to complete the self-assessment in Exhibit 6-2. What are the three major stresses in your life that you have identified?

EXHIBIT 6-2   Holistic Self-Assessment of Stress

Hundreds of surveys and questionnaires are designed to assess one's level of stress. Most, if not all of these, are based on a mechanistic approach to health, not a holistic one (where the whole is considered greater than the sum of parts). The purpose of this self-assessment is to begin to have you look at your problems, issues, and concerns holistically.

1. First, make a list of your current stressors and explain each one:

    1. _____

    2. _____

    3. _____

    4. _____

    5. _____

    6. _____

    7. _____

    8. _____

    9. _____

   10. _____

2. Next, from the list you have just made, reorganize it into acute (short-term) stressors and chronic (prolonged) stressors.

Acute (lasting hours to a few days)	*Chronic (lasting weeks to months)*
1. _____	1. _____
2. _____	2. _____
3. _____	3. _____
4. _____	4. _____
5. _____	5. _____

(continues)

EXHIBIT 6-2   Holistic Self-Assessment of Stress *(continued)*

3. Now, from the first list you made, determine whether each stressor is mental, physical, emotional, or spiritual.

Mental	*Physical*	*Emotional*	*Spiritual*
			Relationships/ values/purpose of life
Overwhelmed/ bored	*Injuries/ sickness*	*Anger or fear based*	
1. _____	1. _____	1. _____	1. _____
2. _____	2. _____	2. _____	2. _____
3. _____	3. _____	3. _____	3. _____
4. _____	4. _____	4. _____	4. _____
5. _____	5. _____	5. _____	5. _____

Source: Brian Luke Seward, PhD (1999). *Managing Stress: Principles and Strategies for Health and Well-Being.* Sudbury, MA: Jones and Bartlett Publishers. Reprinted with permission.

Stress and Disease

As mentioned, the recognition of the link between the mind and the body is not new; however, the specific mechanism to explain the link between stress and disease is still unclear despite years of scientific research. It is widely believed that the impact of stress—especially chronic stress—on the human body greatly increases the risk of developing a variety of diseases such as asthma, arthritis, cancer, hypertension, heart disease, migraine headaches, strokes, and ulcers. Statistics from a variety of sources state that 50–90% of health-related problems are linked to or aggravated by stress.[5,6] Nearly every consumer-oriented publication from hospitals, public health departments, health maintenance organizations, and physician's offices recommends or offers some type of stress-management program.

Most people probably are able to recognize the major physical symptoms of stress in their lives. They also need to be aware of other important behavioral, emotional, or mental symptoms that may be stress related, such as compulsive eating, drinking or smoking, restlessness, irritability or aggressiveness, boredom, inability to focus on the task at hand, trouble thinking clearly, memory loss, or inability to make decisions. The self-assessment tool shown in Exhibit 6-3 contains common physical symptoms often related to stress to help people assess how they are affected by stress in their lives. It is helpful for healthcare professionals to encourage people to engage in a self-assessment as a means to gain insight into

Exhibit 6-3 Stress and Disease: Physical Symptoms Questionnaire

Look over this list of stress-related symptoms and circle how often they have occurred in the past week, how severe they seemed to you, and how long they lasted. Then reflect on the past week's workload and see if you notice any connection.

	How often? (number of days)	How severe? (1 = mild, 5 = severe)	How long? (1 = 1 hour, 5 = all day)
1. Tension headache	0 1 2 3 4 5 6 7	1 2 3 4 5	1 2 3 4 5
2. Migraine headache	0 1 2 3 4 5 6 7	1 2 3 4 5	1 2 3 4 5
3. Muscle tension (neck and/or shoulders)	0 1 2 3 4 5 6 7	1 2 3 4 5	1 2 3 4 5
4. Muscle tension (lower back)	0 1 2 3 4 5 6 7	1 2 3 4 5	1 2 3 4 5
5. Joint pain	0 1 2 3 4 5 6 7	1 2 3 4 5	1 2 3 4 5
6. Cold	0 1 2 3 4 5 6 7	1 2 3 4 5	1 2 3 4 5
7. Flu	0 1 2 3 4 5 6 7	1 2 3 4 5	1 2 3 4 5
8. Stomachache	0 1 2 3 4 5 6 7	1 2 3 4 5	1 2 3 4 5
9. Stomach/abdominal bloating/distention/gas	0 1 2 3 4 5 6 7	1 2 3 4 5	1 2 3 4 5
10. Diarrhea	0 1 2 3 4 5 6 7	1 2 3 4 5	1 2 3 4 5
11. Constipation	0 1 2 3 4 5 6 7	1 2 3 4 5	1 2 3 4 5
12. Ulcer flare-up	0 1 2 3 4 5 6 7	1 2 3 4 5	1 2 3 4 5
13. Asthma attack	0 1 2 3 4 5 6 7	1 2 3 4 5	1 2 3 4 5
14. Allergies	0 1 2 3 4 5 6 7	1 2 3 4 5	1 2 3 4 5
15. Canker/cold sores	0 1 2 3 4 5 6 7	1 2 3 4 5	1 2 3 4 5
16. Dizzy spells	0 1 2 3 4 5 6 7	1 2 3 4 5	1 2 3 4 5
17. Heart palpitations (racing heart)	0 1 2 3 4 5 6 7	1 2 3 4 5	1 2 3 4 5
18. TMJ	0 1 2 3 4 5 6 7	1 2 3 4 5	1 2 3 4 5
19. Insomnia	0 1 2 3 4 5 6 7	1 2 3 4 5	1 2 3 4 5
20. Nightmares	0 1 2 3 4 5 6 7	1 2 3 4 5	1 2 3 4 5
21. Fatigue	0 1 2 3 4 5 6 7	1 2 3 4 5	1 2 3 4 5
22. Hemorrhoids	0 1 2 3 4 5 6 7	1 2 3 4 5	1 2 3 4 5
23. Pimples/acne	0 1 2 3 4 5 6 7	1 2 3 4 5	1 2 3 4 5

(continues)

EXHIBIT 6-3   **Stress and Disease: Physical Symptoms Questionnaire** *(continued)*

	How often? (number of days)	How severe? (1 = mild, 5 = severe)	How long? (1 = 1 hour, 5 = all day)
24. Cramps	0 1 2 3 4 5 6 7	1 2 3 4 5	1 2 3 4 5
25. Frequent accidents	0 1 2 3 4 5 6 7	1 2 3 4 5	1 2 3 4 5
26. Other(please specify)	0 1 2 3 4 5 6 7	1 2 3 4 5	1 2 3 4 5

Score: Look over the entire list. Do you observe any patterns or relationships between your stress levels and your physical health? A value over 30 points may indicate a stress-related health problem. If it seems to you that these symptoms are related to undue stress, they probably are. Although medical treatment is advocated when necessary, the regular use of relaxation techniques may lessen the intensity, frequency, and duration of these episodes.

Source: Brian Luke Seward, PhD (1999). *Managing Stress: Principles and Strategies for Health and Well-Being.* Sudbury, MA: Jones and Bartlett Publishers. Reprinted with permission.

the impact of stress in their lives. This is not only important to maintaining a state of wellness, but also as part of living with chronic conditions.

Stress-Reduction Measures

After people recognize the symptoms of stress in their lives, they can minimize the impact of stress on their physical, mental, emotional, and spiritual well-being by using one or a combination of measures designed for stress reduction. The ultimate goal of stress reduction or stress management is the relaxation response, or a state of profound rest and peace. The term relaxation response was first used by Dr. Herbert Benson in his book of the same name. He cites four elements that are essential to and found in most stress-reduction measures[7]:

1. A quiet environment
2. A mental device, such as a word or a phrase that should be repeated over and over again
3. The adoption of a passive attitude (which is perhaps the most important of the elements)
4. A comfortable position

For purposes of clarification, a *passive attitude* is one in which a person is open to a free flow of thoughts without analysis or judgment.

KEY POINT

Numerous studies of the results of stress reduction have demonstrated positive findings to include the reduction of blood pressure in individuals with hypertension, improved sleeping patterns in individuals suffering from insomnia, decreased nausea and vomiting in chemotherapy patients, and reduction in the multiple symptoms of women diagnosed with premenstrual syndrome or who are experiencing menopausal symptoms.[8]

Individual preferences and circumstances will influence the selection of stress-reduction measures. Some stress-management techniques are simple, whereas others require some initial instruction. Regardless of the choice of method or combination of methods, *all* require practice and need to be used on a regular basis to be effective. Nurses and other healthcare professionals provide a valuable service by instructing, assisting, and coaching people in the use of stress-reduction techniques. Some of the specific measures that can be employed are described in the remainder of this chapter.

Exercise

In the early days of human existence, most threats were physical and demanded an immediate, intense physical response to ensure survival. The response was literally "fight" or "flight." All of the stress hormones released were quickly consumed, and their physical effects were diminished in that burst of activity. In today's environment, the majority of the sources of stress are much less physical and more complex. They usually result from cumulative factors, such as multiple, often simultaneous demands at home and at work.

Physical, emotional, and mental well-being depends on finding a way to dissipate the negative effects of those stressors. Aerobic exercise burns off existing catecholamines and stress hormones by directing them toward their intended metabolic functions, rather than allowing them to linger in the body to undermine the integrity of vital organs. A consistent exercise program has also been demonstrated to help decrease the level of reaction to future stressors. The key to using exercise for stress reduction is to develop an individualized program that is tailored to one's physical abilities, time constraints, and finances. Additionally, selecting an activity that does not increase stress by emphasizing competitiveness rather than relaxation and enjoyment benefits stress reduction.

EXHIBIT 6-4   Progressive Muscular Relaxation Exercise

PMR can be done from a sitting or lying position and usually takes 20–30 minutes to complete. As you take in a deep breath, tighten or tense individual groups of muscles to the count of five. A common sequence to follow is this:

· Forehead	· Shoulders	· Abdomen
· Eyes	· Upper arms	· Pelvis/buttocks
· Jaw	· Lower arms	· Upper legs
· Neck	· Hands	· Lower legs
· Back	· Chest	· Feet

As you focus on each area inhale to the count of five and then exhale slowly, allowing the muscles to relax. Repeat this process twice for each major muscle group or body area.

Progressive Muscular Relaxation

When you are stressed, anxious, angry, or frightened your body automatically responds by increasing muscle tension. You may have experienced the effects of that response resulting in muscular aches and pains in various parts of your body after an unpleasant encounter or a hectic day. Progressive muscular relaxation (PMR) was developed in the 1930s by Dr. Edmund Jacobson, a physician–researcher at the University of Chicago, as a method to reverse this tension and elicit the relaxation response. Moving sequentially from one major muscle group or area of the body to another, for example, from head to toes or vice versa, muscles will be consciously tensed and then relaxed. This conscious muscular activity interrupts the stress response by interfering with the transmission of stress-related tension via the sympathetic nervous system to the muscle fibers.

Among the benefits of PMR are decreases in the body's oxygen use, metabolic rate, respiratory rate, and blood pressure. These effects can have benefits to people diagnosed with hypertension and chronic obstructive lung disease. Additionally, PMR has been shown to be a useful pain management tool in some patients with cancer and chronic pain.[8]

PMR is relatively easy to learn. The method cited in Exhibit 6-4 is only one of the variations on the original technique designed by Dr. Jacobson.

Meditation

Meditation is one of the oldest known techniques for relaxation, dating back to the 6th century BC. There are as many definitions of meditation as there are types of meditation, but basically, it can be understood to be a practice that quiets and relaxes the mind. During a meditative state, the individual strives to let go of all connections to physical senses and conscious thoughts. All focus and awareness is turned inward, with the ultimate goal of calmness and harmony of mind and body. Studies have shown that anxiety, a major symptom of acute stress, was significantly reduced with the regular use of meditation. As stated earlier, there are many techniques for meditation, some with rituals or rules for that specific technique. In *Minding the Body, Mending the Mind*, Joan Borysenko, PhD, presents a simple, eight-step process for meditation that is easily understood[9]:

1. Choose a quiet spot where you will not be disturbed by other people or by the telephone.

2. Sit in a comfortable position.

3. Close your eyes.

4. Relax your muscles sequentially from head to feet.

5. Become aware of your breathing, noticing how the breath goes in and out, without trying to control it in any way.

6. Repeat your focus word silently in time to your breathing.

7. Do not worry about how you are doing.

8. Practice at least once a day for between 10 and 20 minutes.

REFLECTION

Have you built a time for meditation into your daily routine? If not, why? Consider developing a plan to incorporate this practice into your days for the next week. Designate a quiet space. Schedule the time period, and leave yourself a written affirmation (I honor my body, mind, and spirit by taking time to meditate daily). Evaluate your efforts and responses after one week.

Imagery

Imagery is a mental representation of an object, place, event, or situation.[10] In guided imagery, a person is led with specific words, symbols, and ideas to elicit a positive response. People use images regularly when they describe feelings or concepts in their conversations. For example, when stressed, they might say that they feel tied up in knots, or if they receive recognition from an employer for closing a major deal, they may say they feel like they are on top of the world. Those images can convey powerful messages and can be used as a stress-reduction method.

Other Measures

Other measures can be used to help reduce stress, such as music therapy, biofeedback, and diversional activities. Other chapters in this book (herbal remedies [see Chapter 22], aromatherapy [see Chapter 23], and humor [see Chapter 15]) offer additional insights into measures that assist with stress management. It is beneficial for the nurse or other health-care professional to help people understand the dynamics of stress, identify individual sources and responses to stress, develop effective stress-management strategies, and rein-force the significance of efforts to manage stress.

Summary

Hans Selye identified the three stages of stress as the *alarm reaction*, the *stage of resistance*, and the *stage of exhaustion*. Some stress is positive (*eustress*) in that it motivates or has pleasant effects. *Distress* is the bad stress and has negative effects.

The sympathetic nervous system is activated when a person is stressed, which produces many effects in the body. *Psychoneuroimmunology* is the study of the interaction of the mind, the central nervous system, and the immune system and their impact on health.

Identifying and understanding stressors is essential in changing the way stress is managed. Elements of most stress-reduction exercises include a quiet environment, a mental word that can be repeated, adoption of a passive attitude, and a comfortable position. Exercise, meditation, and imagery are among the measures beneficial in stress reduction.

References

1. Selye, H. (1984). *The Stress of Life*. New York: McGraw-Hill, pp. 29–40.
2. Irwin, M., & Vedhara, K. (2005). *Human Psychoneuroimmunology*. New York: Oxford University Press.
3. Seward, B. L. (2005). *Managing Stress: Principles and Strategies for Health and Well-Being*, 5th ed. Sudbury, MA: Jones and Bartlett, p. 5.
4. Girdano, D., Everly, G. S., & Dusek, D. E. (2008). *Controlling Stress and Tension*, 8th ed. Upper Saddle River, NJ: Benjamin Cummings.
5. Seward, B. L. (2005). *Managing Stress: Principles and Strategies for Health and Wellbeing*, 5th ed. Sudbury, MA: Jones and Bartlett.
6. Slade, T. (2007). The descriptive epidemiology of internalizing and externalizing psychiatric dimensions. *Social Psychiatry and Psychiatric Epidemiology. 42*(7):554–560.
7. Benson, H. (2000). *The Relaxation Response*. New York: HarperTorch, p. 110–111.
8. Kwekkeboom, K. L., and Gretasrdottir, E. (2006). Systematic review of relaxation interventions for pain. *Journal of Nursing Scholarship, 38*(3):269–277.
9. Borysenko, J. (2007). *Minding the Body, Mending the Mind*. New York: Bantam Books, pp. 42–46.
10. Post-White, J. (2006). Imagery. In Snyder, M., & Lindquist, R. (eds.). *Complementary/Alternative Therapies in Nursing*. New York: Springer Publishing Company, p. 44.

Suggested Reading

Appel, L. J. (2003). Lifestyle modification as a means to prevent and treat high blood pressure. *Journal of the American Society of Nephrology, 14*(7) (Suppl 2):S99–S102.

Banga, K. (2000). Stress management: a step-by-step process. *Nurse Educator, 25*(3):130, 135.

Bartol, G. M., & Courts, N. F. (2005). The Psychophysiology of Bodymind Healing. In Dossey, B. M., Keegan, L., & Guzetta, C. *Holistic Nursing: A Handbook for Practice*, 3rd ed. Sudbury, MA: Jones and Bartlett, pp. 111–130.

Clark, A. M. (2003). "It's like an explosion in your life": lay perspectives on stress and myocardial infarction. *Journal of Clinical Nursing, 12*(4):544–553.

Davidson, R. J., Kabat-Zinn, J., Schumacher, J., Rosenkranz. M. N., Muller, M., Santorelli,D., et al. (2003). Alterations in brain and immune function produced by mindfulness meditation. *Psychosomatic Medicine, 65*(4):564–570.

Forester, A. (2003). Healing broken hearts. *Journal of Psychosocial Nursing & Mental Health Services, 41*(6):44–49.

Greenberg, J. S. (2006). *Comprehensive Stress Management.* New York: McGraw-Hill.

Haight, B. K., Barba, B. E., Tesh, A. S., & Courts, N. F. (2002). Thriving: a life span theory. *Journal of Gerontological Nursing, 28*(3):14–22.

Jones, M. C., and Johnson, D. W. (2000). Reducing stress in first level and student nurses: a review of the applied stress management literature. *Journal of Advanced Nursing, 32*(1):66–74.

Kenney, J. W. (2000). A women's 'inner balance': a comparison of stressors, personality traits and health problems by age groups. *Journal of Advanced Nursing, 31*(3):639–650.

Lambert V. A., Lambert, C. E., & Yamase, H. (2003). Psychological hardiness, workplace stress and related stress reduction strategies. *Nursing and Health Sciences, 5*(2):181–184.

Mimura, C., & Griffiths, P. (2003). The effectiveness of current approaches to workplace stress management in the nursing profession: an evidence-based literature review. *Occupational & Environmental Medicine, 60*(1):10–15.

Richardson, S. (2003). Effects of relaxation and imagery on the sleep of the critically ill adults. *Dimensions of Critical Care Nursing, 22*(4):182–190.

Seaward, B. L. (2000). *Managing Stress: Principles and Strategies for Health and Well-Being*, 2nd ed. Sudbury, MA: Jones & Bartlett.

Seaward, B. L. (2006). *Stressed Is Desserts Spelled Backwards.* New York: Barnes & Noble Books.

Shealy, C. N. (2002). *90 Days to Stress-Free Living.* Boston: Element Books.

Sloman, R. (2002). Relaxation and imagery for anxiety and depression control in community patients with advanced cancer. *Cancer Nursing, 25*(6):432–435.

Thorpe, K., & Barsky, J. (2001). Healing through self-reflection. *Journal of Advanced Nursing, 35*(5):760–768.

Wheeler, C. M. (2007). *10 Simple Solutions to Stress: How to Tame Tension And Start Enjoying Your Life.* Oakland, CA: New Harbinger Publications.

Yonge, O., Myrick, F., & Hanse, M. (2002). Student nurses' stress in the preceptorship experience. *Nurse Educator, 27*(2):84–88.

Part II

Developing Healthy Lifestyle Practices

Chapter 7

Growing Healthy Relationships

OBJECTIVES

This chapter should enable you to

· Identify the characteristics of a healthy relationship

· Discuss the difference between one's little ego and higher ego

· List four defense mechanisms that people use to protect themselves

· Describe what is meant by a *body memory*

· List at least five personal characteristics that aid in developing healthy relationships

Throughout life, we encounter and form innumerable relationships. Each relationship, no matter how loving or distasteful, how short or long term it may be, contains within it a storehouse of information about our own and others' unique personalities. Each relationship, should we choose to view it with a new openness of mind, offers a rich opportunity to reexamine our innermost selves and to reform, if necessary, the ways in which we perceive and behave in our relationships with other people and in given situations.

But how do we determine healthy versus unhealthy relationships—constructive versus destructive ones? How do relationships become so out of control and out of balance, perhaps to the point of ultimately becoming toxic and disease producing to a person's core being? Precisely what can be done to change these uncomfortable or intolerable relationships in which people tend to find themselves repeatedly?

Identifying Healthy versus Unhealthy Relationships

To begin to answer these questions, we first need to know how to identify a healthy relationship.

KEY POINT

A healthy (human) relationship is one in which there is ongoing mutual trust, respect, caring, honesty, and sharing that is given and received in an environment of nonjudgment and unconditional love and an environment that provides a safe place for physical, mental, emotional, and spiritual growth for all persons involved.

A *healthy relationship* can be defined as "a healthy sense of connection in which two or more persons agree to share hurts, failures, learning, (and) successes in a nonjudgmental fashion (in order) to enhance each other's life potentials."[1] A healthy relationship requires a healthy balance of dependence and healthy independence (see Table 7-1).

In order to form healthier relationships, it is necessary for people to learn about

- Their own unique personalities and idiosyncrasies
- The defensive coping mechanisms they use to react or respond to unconscious or conscious emotions, such as anxiety, anger, fear, conflict, loneliness, envy, and jealousy

This learning *may* best take place in the context of a professional yet trusting relationship with a mental health professional and involve the gradual conscious revealing of previously unrecognized feelings. This process or journey, although at times painful and difficult, can lead to new insights and ways of feeling and being that, perceived through a positive lens, can fill one's life with an expanded consciousness, creating richer meaning and healthier patterns or ways of living and relating to others.

KEY POINT

To take relationships beyond the human sphere, you must also include those you have with yourself, the universe, the planet, animals, your work, your hobbies, material objects (such as money), behaviors (such as eating), smoking, and alcohol consumption; and even the relationships you form with your own bodily illnesses and pain, to mention only a few.

Your Relationship to Self

The most important relationship that you will ever form is the one you create with your true self. This is also the only relationship over which you will ever have any actual or ultimate control. Because the way you relate to your own self significantly impacts how you choose to relate to others, it is imperative, before delving into external or *other* relationships, that you take a look at the meaning of *self* and the inner relationships you have formed with aspects of your many *selves* rooted in your earliest experiences, learning, perceptions, and understanding.

You might think of yourself as consisting of two major selves: your *lower, false self* or *little ego*, and your *authentic, divine self* or *higher ego*. The little ego is the part of you that is dominated and controlled by the emotion of fear. It is the part that creates such feelings as *not good enough, not deserving enough, not smart enough*; all of those "*not enoughs*" prevent you from moving forth to pursue and manifest your dreams. In contrast, your higher ego is defined and directed by the emotion of unconditional love.[2] With your higher ego as your guiding

TABLE 7-1   Tasks in Human Development and Formation of Healthy and Unhealthy Boundaries

Approximate age occurs	Tasks	Healthy boundaries and relationships	Unhealthy boundaries and relationships
Birth to 1 year	Be connected	Infant believes his is part of and extension of parents	Same as healthy
1 year	Trust Feel Love	Mother–infant symbiosis helps organize perceptions and feelings through healthy giving and receiving	Narcissistic or otherwise distracted parents mistreat and mold infant to be an extension of their wants and needs. Parents also may neglect children creating an insecure environment
2 years	Separate Initiate Explore Think	Begins to recognize that he or she is separate from parents; begins to explore world	Parents disallow exploration of world; parents set boundaries that are too rigid or too loose
3 years	Cooperate	Models behaviors and thinking after parents and others who are close	Lack of positive models
4 years	Master	Continues learning how he or she is similar to and different from others	Distortion of sameness into codependence and differentness into low self-esteem
6 years	Evaluate Create Develop morals, skills, values	Continues exploring with growing sense of self	Parents and others stifle healthy exploration and self-esteem
13 years	Evolve Grow	Begins to separate self from parents and family; struggles for further self-identity	Unhealthy separation; distorted boundaries and sense of self
19 years	Develop intimacy	Explores and engages in intimate relationships	Dysfunctional attempts at relationships
Mid- and late-life	Create Extend love Self-actualize Transcend ego	Continued search for God and self; recycles many earlier issues	Spiritual distress; unfulfilled search for God and self

force, you find that you genuinely love yourself and others. This kind of love allows you to believe in yourself and have the confidence that whatever you seek to do or be in life can be envisioned and created in abundance.

REFLECTION

Are there any *not enoughs* that limit you? How do they affect your life?

Love and fear are the two basic emotions from which all other emotions evolve, and it is difficult for these two emotions to coexist within one simultaneously. Unfortunately, many people operate from the perspective of their little ego. They choose to view possibilities as *im*possibilities. Relationships often have an underlying theme of "sure, they like me now, but when they find out who I *really* am, they won't want anything to do with me." Their little ego is deathly afraid of being found out, and thus, they may go about presenting a false face and, consequently, a false self to the world. This classically represents the wisdom of the words "as within, so without." In the fear of confronting and coming to know the true self, they hide it both in their relationship to their inner self and in their outer relationships with others.

KEY POINT

Carl Jung, one of the most renowned and respected psychiatrists of our time, contended that each of our personalities is structurally made up of four archetypes or models and that these archetypes significantly influence our interpersonal behaviors and (therefore) our relationships. His four models include our *persona*, the social mask or face that we reveal to the public, our *shadow*, the parts of ourselves that we disown or deny, our *anima-animus*, the part of us that contains both our male and female characteristics, and our *self*, the part of the personality Jung considered the most significant because it embodies each person's longing for unity and wholeness. Jung also believed that the goal of personality development is self-realization, or as I would interpret this, a remembering, realizing, and reclaiming of our true, authentic self. In our process of seeking and finding our selfhood, Jung proclaimed that we as human beings are transformed from biological creatures into spiritual individuals.[3]

The Search for the Authentic Self

We begin to develop our relationships as infants and young children as we watch and interact with significant people in our lives—parents, siblings, grandparents, extended family and friends, and other authority figures—and to our environment in general. As we grow, we listen, observe, and absorb what is being said and acted out around us. We see how the authority figures in our lives respond and react to different situations and people, and with them as our role models, we tend to embrace the same or similar kinds of patterns in our own lives. If there is a lot of fear and anxiety within the family unit, we may tend to react with that same kind of fear. If there is trust and contentment, our responses, rather than spontaneous defensive reactions, tend to be on a more trusting, calm, and balanced plane. In most families, there will be a mixture of these types of feelings, behaviors, reactions, and responses. Depending on their individual make-ups, people perceive, think, and feel about situations and relationships in their own unique ways.

KEY POINT

Children from the same households with the same parents and circumstances and with very little, if any, notable differences in upbringing are often extremely different personality-wise.

Numerous theories are available as to why individual differences exist. One, not surprisingly, has to do with genetic makeup. One child may "take more" after one side of a family or individual in that family. Another contributing factor is the manner in which one chooses to perceive given events, situations, or people. What one person chooses to take personally and get extremely upset or fearful about, another may take in stride with an attitude of calmness and trust and a certain *knowing* that all will work out as it needs to. If the stimulus in a given situation is overwhelmingly negative, people may develop misperceptions about the world as a whole. They may categorize *all* people as good or bad and *all* situations as either black or white with no gray in between. When young, people are essentially powerless over the circumstances of where and with whom they live. If people are abused or perceive themselves as being wounded in some way, it is natural to look for ways to deny, escape, manipulate, react, or do whatever it takes to ultimately survive in settings that may otherwise be intolerable or literally destructive to their very bodies, minds, souls, and spirits.

Through ages seven or eight, people are much like sponges soaking up whatever is taking place within the world. They have not yet formed any type of protective psychological barrier or screen through which they can filter or sort out the tremendous amount of information and stimuli that is being received. They are left to deal with overwhelmingly negative people, circumstances, and stimuli, with both the good and the bad in life, in the best ways they can manage.

KEY POINT

When adults fail to heal from the wounds of their childhood, there is a strong probability that their wounds will impact their children.

Few people enter adulthood with a totally positive self-esteem. Within most people, there dwells a significant amount of unhealed toxic shame. This shame is the result of low self-esteem born out of painful childhood situations in which people had no ability or permission to choose and during which times their innermost selves felt vulnerable and inappropriately exposed.[2] The psyche was stripped naked. Over and over they may have been told negative things about themselves and even called names that were demeaning. This type of relating from role models cultivated fear and distrust, not only of and for them, but because of the childhood inability to see themselves apart from their role models, it also created fear and distrust within themselves. An individual can grow to literally hate aspects of himself or herself that were identified as the bad, negative, or ugly child. Throughout their lives, until they begin to recognize and heal those self *mis*perceptions, they are doomed to repeat the same words, feel the same feelings, and, in essence, play the same tapes over in their minds that prove to them again and again that they are not good or competent human beings and that no matter what they do it is never enough.

Even if people did not grow up in the worst of circumstances, they face problems and difficulties that require the development of some type of coping strategies. It must be emphasized that in given circumstances, whether what has happened in the past or what is happening in the present is perceived rightly or wrongly, people develop their own unique coping mechanisms that actually work or at least work well at certain times and in given situations.

In the physical realm, people *appear* to be totally separate from others, and given that perception, they naturally form certain defense and coping patterns that serve to act as barriers to anyone or anything that may seem a threat to their well-being; however, from the holistic perspective, there is no such thing as true separation. The body is an energy field that interconnects energetically to others by the vast oceanic universe in which we live.

KEY POINT

Some of the more common defense mechanisms used by people in efforts to protect themselves include *denial, displacement, rationalization, and regression.*

Denial allows people to refuse to see anything that may cause pain or that they don't want or know how to deal with.

Displacement causes people to place blame on other people or situations rather than taking on personal responsibility for whatever is happening in their lives.

Rationalizations are simply mental justifications for the inappropriate actions, feelings, and thoughts people have.

Regression is a reverting back to more primitive or childish behaviors, such as whining, pouting, yelling, cursing, and even physical hitting or beatings. It occurs when feeling out of control and is connected to feelings of loss of control or power.

These unhealthy coping mechanisms, along with a large score of others, are fear based and create barriers between people that block the ability to form loving, intimate relationships.

Intimacy versus Isolation, Love versus Fear

The coping mechanisms that people develop, as noted previously, may have helped them to survive the otherwise intolerable times in their lives. It is only later, when they are older and free from a toxic family and/or environment, that they may undergo an "ah-ha" experience. At this time, they realize that these particular ways of relating, these old patterns of behavior, are simply not working for them any longer. They may feel a desperate need to change, to relate differently, but they simply do not know how.

KEY POINT

Old patterns of thinking and behaving can become so entrenched, so much a part of who a person is, that even the *suggestion* of change can feel too overwhelming, frightening, and threatening.

The process of change can feel as though some sort of death is occurring. In a very real sense, this is true. Even though people are not *really* dying—they actually are healing and transforming old parts of themselves—but the very act of moving through that incredible process can feel extremely scary. Any time people go from what is familiar and "fits like an old shoe" and metaphorically step into a new pair of shoes representing a new, unknown, and unfamiliar world, their natural human instinct is to resist. Intellectually, they may realize that the changes they are choosing to make are all in their own best interest. Still, their emotional tendency is to hold tight to what has felt right for such a long time.

It is at times such as these that the soul is searching to find what has been missing from life all along. People begin to develop an awareness that there are others who appear to have something missing from them. That something, although it may not be easily identified or defined right away, is the ability to love and form intimate relationships without the anxiety and fear of rejection or abandonment.

REFLECTION

Intimacy is the ability to form close or intense (as in marriage) relationships in which you share your life easily and openly with others who have also developed this capacity. With whom do you share intimate relationships? Are they satisfying? Nurturing?

Intimate relationships do not have to be limited to other humans. People can form them with pets, certain causes that they support, or their creative efforts. When we think about marriage or any relationship akin to a lifelong partnership between two people, intimacy grows out of the capacity these two people have for mutual love and their ability to pledge a total commitment to each other. This intimacy goes far beyond any sexual relationship they may have. Rather than a person, this type of commitment could be formed with a particular career, cause, or endeavor that one chooses to devote his or her life. No matter with whom or what one decides to become intimately involved, personal sacrifices will be made in the giving of self. The ability for this kind of intimacy is learned when, as children, people have been the recipients of unconditional love, nurturing and sharing within their family unit.

The inability to form intimate relationships results in withdrawal, social isolation, and loneliness. People may seek what they think is intimacy through numerous superficial friendships or sexual contacts. No career is established; instead, they may have a history of job changes, or they may so fear change that they remain most or all of their adult lives in undesirable job situations.

Body Memories as Blocked Manifestations of Relating

In the holistic framework, your body does not end with your skin. Surrounding you are mental, emotional, and spiritual subtle bodies that are invisible to the average human eye. These bodies are sometimes referred to as *auras* and are reported to be seen by certain people who are sensitive to that particular energy. When all of these bodies are in harmony, both with your internal and external worlds, there is a constant circulating free flow of energy; however, when that balance is disturbed and the energy is blocked on one or more levels, you experience imbalance and disharmony. Left unattended and untreated, the imbalance eventually leads to discomfort and/or disease on all levels. These energetic "holding patterns," or *body memories* (events stored within the physical body at the cellular level), can be and often are, literally *stuck* emotions within your physical, mental, emotional, and/or spiritual bodies. These memories may be of a pleasant or unpleasant quality, of a conscious or unconscious nature. Illness can result from disharmony among these various aspects of the self, reinforcing the importance of addressing body, mind, emotions, and spirit to affect healing.

Every relationship encountered, be it with a friend or perceived foe, brings back a part of self that was missing. When that part resonates within, it is transformative, drawing a person closer to wholeness. Healing seldom, if ever, occurs in a vacuum. Healing does not involve or affect just one person. Rather, people are continually, whether knowingly or unknowingly, consciously or unconsciously, participating together as copartners in healing—in their relationships with others and their relationship with the planet and a higher power.

The Role of Forgiveness in Relationships

He drew a circle that shut me out—
Heretic, rebel, a thing to flout.
But love and I had a way to win:
We drew a circle that took him in.

UNKNOWN

Perhaps more than any other quality in your life, the ability to forgive is the key to inner peace. Mentally, spiritually, and emotionally, it transforms fear into love. Many times the perceptions of other people and situations become a battleground between the ego, or the lesser self's desire to judge and find fault, whereas the higher authentic self desires to accept people as they are. The lesser ego is a relentless fault finder in both self and others; however, the places in which a person estranges from love are not faults, but wounds. The authentic self seeks out its innocence and never seeks to punish, but rather to heal self and others.

Why, a person might ask, would I *not* judge or find fault with something I know to be wrong? The emphasis here needs to be placed on the behavior or the action as opposed to the person. When one perceives the action and the person as the same, it is impossible to see the person as innocent and his or her actions as unhealed wounds.

KEY POINT

Forgiveness is selective remembering—a conscious decision to focus on love and let the rest go.[4] It is easy to forgive those who have never done anything to make you seriously upset or angry; however, it is the people who trigger you, who push your buttons, who create fear and self-doubt, who are your best teachers. They measure your capacity to love unconditionally, and it is this very love that brings healing to all the lives involved, including your own.

Personal Characteristics in the Development of Healthy Relationships

Dorothea Hover-Kramer[1] has identified eight major personal characteristics that can be tremendously helpful in developing healthy relationships. The following is a modification of her list:

1. Being willing to take a genuine look at one's own faulty personal defenses and blind spots and begin the process of identifying and letting go of these defense patterns

2. Creating a correct sense of self-worth, confidence, and self-esteem; having no grandiosity, yet not putting oneself down

3. Developing flexibility; looking at people and situations from different perspectives; a willingness to "walk in another's shoes"

4. Developing a willingness to take personal responsibility for all of one's feelings or actions

5. Setting conscious awareness of one's spiritual essence and wholeness experienced as a sacred space of inner calm, and setting boundaries that allow for a clear sense of purpose, goal orientation, and direction

6. Making the effort to be understood, persevering to find common ground; seeking and integrating (genuinely taking in) feedback

7. Developing sincere empathy and mutual respect for others without appeasing, complying, or attempting to be overly pleasing

8. Committing oneself to a willingness to revisit, rethink, and redefine previous decisions; accepting the possibility of being wrong and allowing others the space to acknowledge their mistakes

These are characteristics that can be easily identified in effective communicators and negotiators. They bring integrity and balance to the art and skill of successful communication, which is necessary to the building, maintenance, and enhancement of healthy relationships.

The suggestions for having, maintaining, and growing healthy relationships that have been discussed in this chapter correlate to many of the principles that Deepak Chopra has promoted in his writing and teaching.[5] Chopra strongly emphasizes that success is a journey, not a destination and you should never expect to "arrive," and that you will continue throughout your life to learn and hopefully grow from your experiences. He suggests that a basic need that people have to build healthy relationships is for daily *stillness*—meditation or prayer time during which they can go within and listen to the silence from which comes the wisdom of their spiritual and innermost beings. It is through this silence that they ultimately get in touch with their ability to heal old faulty ways of thinking and behaving, to manifest and create their bliss, and it is also through this practice that, over time, they come to realize that low self-esteem (relationship to self) combined with a large dose of fear and negative thinking are the only barriers between themselves and what they desire most in life.

Giving is another crucial ingredient for successful relationships. What is given does not have to be extraordinary, but it does have to be genuine. It may take time, energy, and monies that could be spent elsewhere and experiencing life as more pleasant and less demanding in that moment. This type of giving does not demand nor expect anything in return and is given in the spirit of unconditional love.

Receiving can be the hardest for many people. If people grew up never feeling worthy or deserving, then accepting anything given freely to them by others can be most difficult. In order to grow, they need to have the ability to receive. Chopra notes that it is helpful to affirm oneself with such thoughts as, "Today I will gratefully receive all the gifts that life has to offer me, including the gifts of sunlight, birds singing, spring showers, or the first snow of winter. I will be open to receiving from others and will make a commitment to keep (positive relationships) circulating in my life by giving and receiving life's most precious gifts: the gifts of caring, affection, appreciation, and love."[6]

Next comes acute awareness of the choices made in each moment and how, in the mere witnessing of these choices, they are brought into conscious realization. One begins to understand that the best way to prepare for any future moment is to be fully conscious in the present.

Acceptance of people, situations, circumstances, and events as they occur is another key part of fully entering into a state of peace with self, others, and the world. One can know that the moment is as it should be and consciously choose not to struggle against what cannot be changed.

KEY POINT

When people accept, they take *responsibility* for problems, choosing not to blame anyone or anything (including themselves) for what is happening. Rather, they recognize all events and situations as opportunities in disguise . . . opportunities that they can take and transform into a greater benefit for all involved.

Defenselessness is another important component, according to Chopra. People must let go of the need to defend their point of view. The need to persuade or convince others to accept a point of view is a use of energy that could be much better spent elsewhere. Remaining open to all points of view and not rigidly attaching to any one of them allow for a plethora of choices and opportunities that people may have been blind to within their defensiveness.

Detachment is the last ingredient. Detachment, he says, allows an individual and others the freedom to be who they are and to travel their life paths as they must while remaining unattached to the outcome. This detachment does not mean that people do not care. In contrast, they deeply care and are concerned about those with whom they relate, and they are there for others in loving, caring ways. Once again, however, they must not interfere or try to do others' processes for them. People must learn in their own way and at their own pace what feels right for them. They may have later come to the conclusion that a person who gave them advice was right all along, but what is significant is that they chose to act on it in their own time and at their own pace.

REFLECTION

Do you tend to force your opinions and advice on others when you are confident that you know what is in their best interest? If you think for just a moment about how resentful and angry you felt when others have attempted to take over or force your choices in a particular direction, it does not take long to see how your attempts to do the same with others can so easily backfire.

As people begin to understand and absorb the principles Chopra outlines, they can gradually unblock painful and disease-producing energy that has been kept in and, in doing so, allow that energy to become more balanced and free flowing. This action frees them to discover their unique talents and to create and manifest long-held dreams. At the same time, they also are freed up to serve and respond to others with an unconditional and unbounded love.

In this global, multicultural world, people are continually encountering a wide variety of people from different cultures, beliefs, backgrounds, skills, and education. Access to advanced technology through the Internet and other avenues has given people the means to bring different parts of the world right into their own homes. In doing so, they are forced to a greater extent than ever before, to deal with other people, cultures, ideas, information, and beliefs that may be profoundly different from their own; however, if individuals are willing to crack the door to the possibility of experiencing a new consciousness, they can begin the step forward toward the creation of richer, healthier relationships and lives filled with an abundance of experiences, learning, and growth that previously would have been unimaginable.

Summary

A healthy relationship is one in which there is ongoing mutual trust, respect, caring, honesty, and sharing that is exchanged in an environment of nonjudgment and unconditional love. Learning about oneself fosters the building of healthy relationships.

Healthy relationships are not built on neediness, but on love and caring. Major personal characteristics are helpful in developing healthy relationships, such as a willingness to look at oneself honestly, creating a realistic sense of self-worth, having flexibility, being aware of spiritual essence, making an effort to be understood, having empathy and respect for others, and acknowledging one's own mistakes.

Deepak Chopra describes the requirements for successful relationships, which include the need for stillness, giving, receiving, awareness of choices, acceptance of people and circumstances, defenselessness, and detachment. With an understanding of these principles, people can gradually unblock painful and disease-producing energy that has been long held within and be freed to serve and respond to others with an unconditional and unbounded love.

References

1. Hover-Kramer, D. (2004). Relationships. In Dossey, B. M., Keegan, L., & Guzzetta, C. E. (eds.). *Holistic Nursing: A Handbook for Practice*, 4th ed. Sudbury, MA: Jones and Bartlett, p. 670.
2. Bradshaw, J. (2005). *Healing the Shame That Binds You*. Deerfield Beach, FL: Health Communications, Inc.
3. Jung, C. G. (2006). *The Undiscovered Self*. New York: New American Press.
4. Williamson, M. (2005). *A Return to Love: Reflections on the Principles of a Course in Miracles*. New York: HarperCollins.
5. Chopra, D. (2007). *The Seven Spiritual Laws of Success: A Practical Guide to the Fulfillment of Your Dreams*. San Rafael, CA: co-published by Amber-Allen Publishing and New World Library, p. 2.

6. Chopra, D. (2007). *The Seven Spiritual Laws of Success: A Practical Guide to the Fulfillment of Your Dreams.* San Rafael, CA: co-published by Amber-Allen Publishing and New World Library, p. 36.

Suggested Reading

Autry, J. A. (2002). *The Spirit of Retirement. Creating a Life of Meaning and Personal Growth.* New York: Prima Press.

Barnum, B. S. (2003). *Spirituality in Nursing,* 2nd ed. New York: Springer Publishing Company.

Bender, M., Bauchham, P., & Norris, A. (1999). *The Therapeutic Purpose of Reminiscence.* Thousand Oaks, CA: Sage.

Borysenko, J. (1998). *A Woman's Book of Life: The Biology, Psychology, and Spirituality of the Feminine Life Cycle.* New York: Riverhead Books.

Carson, V. B., and Arnold, E. N. (eds.). (2000). *Mental Health Nursing: The Nurse-Patient Journey,* 2nd ed. Philadelphia: W. B. Saunders & Co.

Carter-Scott, C. (2000). *If Life Is a Game, These Are the Rules.* New York: Broadway Books.

Cox, A. M., & Albert, D. H. (2003). *The Healing Heart: Communities.* Gabriola Island, Canada: New Society Publishers.

Felton, B. S., & Hall, J. M. (2001). Conceptualizing resilience in women older than 85: overcoming adversity from illness or loss. *Journal of Gerontological Nursing, 27*(11):46–53.

Hertz, J. E., & Anschutz, C. A. (2002). Relationships among perceived enactment of autonomy, self-care, and holistic health in community dwelling older adults. *Journal of Holistic Nursing, 20*(2):166–186.

Hillman, J. (2000). *The Force of Character and the Lasting Life.* New York: Random House.

Lemme, B. H. (2005). *Development in Adulthood,* 4th ed. Boston: Allyn & Bacon.

Moore, S. L., Metcalf, B., & Schow, E. (2000). Aging and meaning in life: examining the concept. *Geriatric Nursing, 21*(1):27–29.

Puentes, W. J. (2000). Using social reminiscence to teach therapeutic communication skills. *Geriatric Nursing, 21*(3):318–320.

Quadagno, J. S. (2007). *Aging and the Life Course: An Introduction to Social Gerontology.* Boston: McGraw-Hill College.

Semmelroth, C. (2002). *The Anger Habit Workbook. Proven Principles to Calm the Stormy Mind.* Calrsbad, CA: Writers Club Press.

Snowden, D. (2002). *Aging with Grace: What the Nun Study Teaches us about Leading Longer, Healthier, and More Meaningful Lives.* New York: Random House.

Thomas, E. L., & Eisenhandler, S. A. (1999). *Religion, Belief, and Spirituality in Late Life.* New York: Springer.

Wallace, S. (2000). Rx RN: A Spiritual approach to aging. *Alternative and Complementary Therapies, 6*(1):47–48.

Wilt, D. L., & Smucker, C. J. (2001). *Nursing the Spirit.* Washington, DC: American Nurses Publishing.

Wolf, T. P. (2003). Building a caring client relationship and creating a quilt. a parallel and metaphorical process. *Journal of Holistic Nursing, 21*(1):81–87.

Chapter 8

Survival Skills for Families

OBJECTIVES

This chapter should enable you to

- List at least five types of families
- Describe at least three assumptions about families
- Discuss the body, mind, and spirit of a family
- Outline at least six questions that can be used to explore the balance of work and family needs
- Describe seven major components of a Healthy Options Assessment
- List the six steps of goal setting
- Describe what is meant by holistic parenting

Family is a word that represents something very personal, yet common, to each of us. There was a time when the word family conjured up an image of a husband, wife, and dependent children; however, recent decades have revised this image as a result of relaxed sexual mores, increased acceptance of alternate lifestyles, the women's movement, and other factors. Families take a variety of forms:

- Blended families
- Single-parent families
- Families with one child
- Families with many children
- Same-gender partner families
- Grandparents raising grandchildren
- Young parent families
- Older parent families
- Couples without children

These families can be youthful or seasoned, multigenerational, legally married, or partnered without the benefit of marriage. With these changes have come less clear rules and boundaries in the way families behave.

REFLECTION

What meaning does family hold for you? Examining your personal beliefs about the meaning of family and the cultural and social influences that surround family is one step toward developing successful survival skills as a family.

Just as there is a cultural evolution redefining the description of family, there is a personal one as well. Each family changes with time. Even with the same people and the same composition individual family members age, develop new interests, gain new friends, move to other communities, or change jobs. Each change that happens to one person within a family has an affect on the whole. Accepting and acting on this principle of holism is a step toward developing successful survival skills for families.

KEY POINT

Each family

· Is unique in its beliefs, identity, composition, gifts, and challenges
· Influences and is influenced by its community and its culture
· Shares many things in common with other families
· Deserves respect and opportunities to be successful
· Has the responsibility to respect and care for each of its members while accepting each person as an individual and encouraging their personal health and growth

Family Identity

What's in a name? That which we call a rose,
By any other name would smell as sweet.

WILLIAM SHAKESPEARE, *ROMEO AND JULIET*

When was the last time you looked at your birth certificate? Among the spaces that include the date, time, and place of your birth are the spaces for your mother's maiden name and your father's name. This record of birth, completed or not, forms part of your identity. You are far more than a piece of paper, yet this document follows you through life and represents your heritage.

What meaning do those names hold for you? Were you named after someone, living or deceased? Do you have a middle name? Are you called by the name inscribed there, or over the years have you gained and lost nicknames? Did any of those nicknames stick and become the name to which you now respond?

The names on a birth certificate may give a clear picture of the origins of a family going back to the "old country." Perhaps names have been altered to fit the late 19th century view of what it meant to be an American. Somewhere in the dusty stacks of a family's history are the storytellers who know. They carry the tales and the details of where a family originated and how long a family has been in this country. There are the tales of courage of those who traveled, learned a new language, received an education, and raised a large, successful family. When one stops to think about it, the challenges faced by ancestors are amazing.

Even when the stories are shadows or memories created from a need to know more about family background, people gain an appreciation for the courage and life of their ancestors that brought them here and gave them life. Those names and stories, whether clear or hazy, contribute to their identity and that of their family.

REFLECTION SUNDAY DINNER: A GUIDED REFLECTION

How far back in your childhood can you remember? Were you 2, 3, or 4 years old? If someone asked you to talk about Sunday dinner when you were 10, how would you respond? You may have clear memories of special foods, aromas, the time of day, your place at the table, who was present, and who was not. In your family, who prepared the meal, set the table, cleared the dishes, cleaned up? Compare that with your Sunday dinner last week. Answer the same questions. Are there similarities between Sunday dinner then and now? What were the differences? Ask each adult in your family to reflect on those similarities and the differences, then and now.

What does identity have to do with balancing family, work, and leisure? Balance—be it on ice skates, a bicycle, or juggling the many needs and desires of a family—happens when people know where they are in space; they have focus, and they understand their purpose. They know who they are, where they have come from, and where they are headed.

KEY POINT

One interesting dynamic about families is that each represents a merging of the identity, needs, and desires of two or more people. People may be different as individuals, but when joined together as a family, their success depends in part on their ability to develop a unique definition of family that all members can accept and value. Finding and maintaining a balance between the needs of the family and those of each individual member contribute to a family's survival skills.

Family identity is based on many things and may change over time; as individuals mature, children leave the nest, and life presents new opportunities, challenges, and surprises. This identity is reflected in where families live, what foods they prefer, religious or spiritual beliefs, political values, lifestyle preferences, educational interests, and vocational choices. It can include their rest/activity patterns, favored forms of entertainment and recreation, and the nature of their personal relationships.

Articulating family identity requires people to sit in peace and equality, each as individuals contributing to the family unit. Each person brings together what he or she desires personally and what each is able to contribute to the whole.

Exhibit 8-1 offers a Family Identity Exercise. It could be beneficial for you to complete this yourself before using it with others. As you complete this exercise, focus on your family and what is needed for its health and success while acknowledging each person's need for respect and opportunities for growth. Maintaining such a focus contributes to the holistic awareness of your family's unique composition. As you proceed with this exercise, think in terms of body, mind, and spirit.

The body of the family describes the physical connection—how they are joined genetically, legally, and emotionally. Body acknowledges how things get done within the system: the responsibilities of childcare, transportation, home maintenance, meal preparation, financial management, and the myriad daily things a family has to do.

Mind includes the common belief systems and how the family thinks, reviews the past, plans for the future, and adjusts to life through learning. Mind touches on the many realms of human life; it influences communication and relationships and the ability to adapt to change.

Spirit acknowledges the awareness that there is something beyond the here and now. Some families manifest their spirituality by adopting a specific lifestyle; others do so through their religions or by contributing to their communities. Still, others define themselves as perpetual seekers, seeking an intense "something" that links them to others beyond the family.

As families explore their unique connections with and contributions to the whole, words and practices may become apparent that help to clarify a family's unique expression of their spirituality. Defining that which is meaningful from the heart and uplifting in daily life supports a family's sense of spirit.

As you go through this exercise, think of key words and phrases to describe your family in selected categories. Under *Food Choices*, a family that has some vegetarian members, whereas others eat meat may describe themselves as being mixed or varied. This description acknowledges that variety and choice are welcome. Their food choice statement might mention that "variety is the spice of life" and then go on to list favorite menus.

A family that limits use of technology by using television or radio only for special broadcasts could include the word *selective* in their media use description. Those who read newspapers, magazines, and journals can find words or phrases that reflect their reading style. Their identity may be varied, reflective of popular culture, or aligned with their recreational interests.

EXHIBIT 8-1   Family Identity Exercise

The following categories of body, mind, and spirit include topics to think about and discuss in relation to your family's identity. These lists can be lengthened or shortened. The purpose is to stimulate conversation about who you are and who you want to be as a family. Try reviewing them as a family unit.

Body

Type of area where you live (country, city, suburbs; region of the nation): _____

_____

Your dwelling place is a(n) (apartment, condominium, house, ranch): _____

_____

Your food preferences are: _____

_____

Your physical recreation is: _____

Your overall health is: _____

You receive your health care from: _____

You describe your financial situation as being: _____

Mind

Your educational achievements include: _____

Your educational interests and goals for your children (if applicable) include: _____

_____

Your reading interests, individually, and as a family are: _____

_____

The forms of arts and entertainment you enjoy are: _____

You use these types of media and technology: _____

_____

Your political preference is: _____

Voting habits of adults in the family are: _____

Your favorite topics of conversation are: _____

_____

Favorite activities that nurture your creativity include: _____

_____

You participate in the following groups and community activities: _____

_____

Spirit

Traditions, rituals, and spiritual practices that are honored by your family include: _____

_____

(continues)

Exhibit 8-1 Family Identity Exercise *(continued)*

You realize meaning and purpose in your life through: _____

_____

Your religious preference, if any, is: _____

You intentionally engage with nature in these ways: _____

_____

You consider the following volunteer activities to be part of your spiritual experience:

_____

People who are very dear to you include: _____

_____

_____

_____

You will notice that some areas overlap. This is holism at work; those topics that thread between body, mind, and spirit are supporting wholeness within your family's life. A family who lives in the country, reads magazines focused on country living, and spends leisure time outdoors feels very much a part of the natural world. Their identity with nature is strong and influences the choices they make throughout their lives.

As you complete and reflect on the Family Identity Exercise, think about your current situation and what you want for the future. The family in the country may be longing for a move to the city. They want more social diversity and a greater variety of arts and entertainment right at their doorstep. Those who live in the city may wish for the peace and open space of the country. Such interests have the potential to determine choices they will make in their work, dwelling place, and community activities.

The descriptions chosen in the Family Identity Exercise will offer guidance in determining how to achieve balance between family, work, and leisure.

Family and Work

Work for most families is a necessity. Livelihood is literally our bread and butter, the means for the roofs over our heads. For some, work or career becomes an expression of who they are. A person's job can affect the family, and in turn, family needs may affect the job.

Creating balance between work and family occurs in an atmosphere of mutual respect. There are workplaces that are family friendly, offering flexible hours, health insurance, vacation hours, childcare benefits, and employee-assistance programs. The best employers are understanding of families while having reasonable work expectations.

When the family is respectful of the work of its members, people are able to be punctual, have good attendance, and maintain focus while at work. Consistency in these areas should mean that an employee is treated courteously when they are then called away for family needs.

Salary or hourly wages are important but may not account for the most desirable aspects of a job. Questions that explore how work life aligns with your family life are offered in Exhibit 8-2.

Creating a balance between work and family responsibilities can be achieved, even partially, by having a clear understanding of the needs and limitations of each. After these are established it is important to convey your limits to both family and work. Sample statements are these:

- "I'll be able to go on your field trip if I get approval from my supervisor."
- "I'm available to attend one evening meeting three weeks a month. I'll need to check with my family if I'm requested to work extra evenings."
- "I prefer flexing my hours to working overtime."
- "I'll be working a little late on Thursday and would like to have supper ready when I get home at 7:30."

While following guidelines such as these, it is advisable for people to know and understand their employee rights and obligations. An employer's attitude toward family and flex-

---

Exhibit 8-2   Exploring Work and Family Needs

1. Do the hours of business create a reasonable match for family responsibilities and desires?

2. What benefits, written and unwritten, are provided to employees at various pay levels?

3. Is there flexibility in where I do my work? Am I able to work at home when my child has a day off from school?

4. Is the employer one that meets or exceeds the conditions of the federal government's Family and Medical Leave Act?

5. Is my workplace a reasonable commute from home?

6. Is my workplace free of hazards, and does it actively promote staff health and safety?

7. Is there support for continuing education with both allocation of time and financial reimbursement?

8. Is there a wage and benefits package that allows me to provide for my family as I wish?

9. Is this a workplace and job that supports my personal and family values and beliefs?

10. Does this workplace embrace employee suggestions and involvement?

11. Are customers of this business viewed holistically and with respect and dignity?

ibility can vary over time or with a change in supervisors. Ultimately, it is the responsibility of the individual employee to know the employer's limitations and to advocate for change if warranted.

Another point to consider in balancing family and work is that each family/work scenario is unique. What works for one family may not work for another. Part-time employment may not have exciting financial benefits but may provide the time to become more involved in a child's activities and education. The family as a whole can determine the best mix for their current situation. When circumstances change, family/work balance can be re-evaluated and new combinations developed as desired. Exhibit 8-3 lists questions that can guide families in exploring these issues.

Families and Leisure

Leisure is defined as freedom from the demands of work or duty free.[1] Families today are very much on the go, continually on the move, around town and across the country. Everyone has much to do—responsibilities to home and family, a job or career, and health and fitness. When and how can anyone plan for fun? With all that needs to be accomplished, how can leisure happen?

People have busy lives, and thus, creating leisure, whether personal or for the family, often requires planning. Spontaneity would be wonderful fun, but it often does not fit in with the structure of the average life.

EXHIBIT 8-3 Questions to Reflect on Regarding Yourself, Your Family, and Family Roles in Relation to Work

· What days and hours do I want or need to be home with my family? Are there certain times of day that I want to be available for them?

· Does my family understand my profession/career/job and its responsibilities?

· What messages do I convey to my family about my workplace, my career, and my work-related goals?

· Do I/we have backup plans for childcare, transportation, and illness?

· Who assumes the responsibilities for chores, meal preparation, and family coordination? Are household and family tasks shared cooperatively?

· Do I foresee that I will need to plan for family changes over the coming years? These may include the needs of dependent adults or a change in the number and ages of children.

· Are there established ground rules related to my work? Examples include accepting phone calls or leaving during business hours for family appointments and activities.

REFLECTION

Say the words *unhurried ease* aloud three times, and say them slowly. What sorts of images arise for you: time to smell the roses, ladies twirling parasols in a green-grassed Monet, the sweet schuss of powdered snow beneath skis? As your imagination creates more pictures of what you would do with free time, what you would do with unhurried ease, shift to your body. Has your breathing relaxed? Have your muscles softened? Hopefully the answer to these questions is yes. If so, you are experiencing the importance of leisure. Daydreaming, spacing out, doing nothing, taking a nap, and taking your time are simple yet important acts that are a forgotten art for many. Wildlife and animals are excellent models for how to enjoy each moment, time to live with unhurried ease. Observe the bird as it perches to preen its feathers, a cat lounging in the afternoon sun, a moose and her young browsing on rich swamp delicacies.

Making a commitment to leisure is making a commitment to oneself. Relaxation is a practice, as are playing the piano, meditating, and woodworking. Daily practice encourages people to become skilled and proficient in the art of leisure and relaxation. By pausing, even for a brief moment, during the busiest days to focus on breath, an individual takes the time to renew.

KEY POINT

In their book *Everyday Blessings*, Myla and Jon Kabat Zinn[2] remind us that mindfulness means moment-to-moment, nonjudgmental awareness. It is cultivated by refining our capacity to pay attention, intentionally, in the present moment, and then sustaining that attention over time as best we can. In the process, we become more in touch with our lives as they are unfolding.

A family commitment to leisure acknowledges that needs related to free time varies from one person to another. Quiet contemplation is meaningful to one while creating garden space is the height of joy for another. Rock music and rock climbing may symbolize unhurried ease to some, but not to others.

Ideally, a plan to create balance through leisure includes individual as well as family relaxation periods. Scheduling unstructured family time works because it affirms commitment to self and the family unit. When a block of time is set aside for family, individual members can go with the flow or plan an activity that has group meaning. They may go somewhere for hours or days or stay at home and plan something out of the ordinary. The key is to remain focused on their together time and to avoid old patterns of distraction.

Some families set aside a family day, a time to be together, exceptions occurring only for special reasons or occasions. This form of structure opens the way for group leisure and time together that can lead to spontaneous moments such as a cookout, a walk in the park, or a drive to the shore. Families can be encouraged to make a wish list of activities to do with unhurried ease and tailor it to the moment.

> **REFLECTION**
>
> As you think about leisure and how to use it to create balance in your life, go back to your family identity descriptions. Who are you now as a family? Are there ways in which you want to change? Do you see where leisure will enhance your overall well-being, uplifting your spirit while moving your body and quieting your mind?

As people take steps toward creating balance between family, work, and leisure, they will begin to note shifts in their behaviors or in those of others around them. It becomes easier to say no to extra duties . . . anywhere. Sunsets last longer. They do learn to focus on their breath. They do share a kiss and hug when leaving for work. The roses somehow do smell sweeter than they did in the past.

Healthy Habits for Families

Habits are patterns of behavior. They are established or discarded over time and with practice. After habits are firmly in place, they can be hard to change because people act almost without thinking. Recall the time when seat belts first came into use. Many would forget to wear them, buckling up only after a friendly reminder from the car itself or from a fellow passenger. Fastening a seat belt is now as automatic as starting the car.

Decision-making and choices enter into this topic area as well. How do people decide when it is time to adopt one behavior over another? Is it an area in which they feel free to choose, or does it tend to result from the suggestion of another person? Are they choosing this habit because they were told it would be good for them or because it is something they believe in and embrace with a full heart? Is it something they are trying for someone else's benefit in hopes that it will improve their relationship? Is the habit they are adopting healthy for their entire family, and have they been respectful of others' needs while seeking to meet their own?

The discussion of healthy habits for families will align with and build on the Family Identity Exercise. Comments and thoughts summarized in this activity will help to assess if current habits or those being sought contribute to the family's individuality, thereby promoting overall health.

Body includes where people live, their type of dwelling, food choices, physical activity, and finances. These are the most basic needs: to have food and shelter and the ability to pay for them. People need to be able to physically move from one place to another and may depend on others or physical means to do so.

EXHIBIT 8-4   How Does Your Community's Profile Contribute or Detract from Your Family's Identity, Goals, and Well-Being?

· Environment/climate/geography

· Population density

· Overall safety

· Infrastructure: roads, government, utilities, transportation, and fire/police/rescue

· Service base: education, health care, and social services

· Spiritual life/civic organizations

· Recreation/arts/cultural events

· Employment options/economic base/sustainability

· Tax base

· Overall quality of life/acceptance of diversity

The city or town in which they live and the dwelling in which they reside can help to promote family identity and the life people choose to lead. They may find that their neighborhood has some limitations or influences that are unhealthy for what they want in their lives. Exhibit 8-4 depicts the numerous elements of country, city, or village life to consider when assessing the current or future situation. As each item is reviewed, evaluate how the community contributes to or detracts from the family's identity, goals, and well-being.

When considering a move in the future, a family should consider its dream town. The qualities that are most important for the family's health and well-being need to be prioritized and used as a guide for their search.

The sense of place is then moved from a community focus to a family focus. This includes household members and home. Families need to think about the living space, both common areas and private areas. Does the home provide designated places for people to gather for meals and conversation? Does it assure that people have rooms or corners to call their own? Even in crowded situations, the surroundings can be adapted by consciously choosing behaviors that contribute to privacy. To do so is respectful because expectations are clarified about space, times for bathing, quiet hours, and meals.

Healthy Options

Attending to their relationships while planning for privacy contributes to the manner in which family members nurture or nourish each other. The topic of nourishment includes providing for the mind and spirit as well as feeding the body. Each statement in the Healthy Options Assessment (see Exhibit 8-5) represents the behaviors and practices of families

---

EXHIBIT 8-5   Healthy Options Assessment

Consider the following nourishment statements, and note your level of agreement (most of the time, sometimes, or rarely) with each. This activity is not intended to be scored or to rate you on your abilities; the purpose is to determine your family's individual patterns and establish if there are changes you would like to make.

	Most of the time	Sometimes	Rarely
A. Food			
· We are satisfied with our diet and believe that it is healthy.	____	____	____
· We eat together as a family every day.	____	____	____
· We eat our meals at the table.	____	____	____
· We eat without distractions such as television.	____	____	____
· We honor each other's food choices.	____	____	____
· We limit our use of stimulating or depressing substances.	____	____	____
B. Communication and Displays of Affection			
· We communicate about our schedules (work, games, meetings, etc.).	____	____	____
· We routinely check in with each other by phone, notes, or e-mail.	____	____	____
· We support each other with positive statements.	____	____	____
· We each have opportunities to express our opinions.	____	____	____
· We use hugs, kisses, and healthy touch to communicate with each other.	____	____	____
· We use and practice effective listening skills.	____	____	____
· We practice the arts of apology and forgiveness.	____	____	____
C. Physical Activity			
· We exercise 3 to 5 times a week for at least 20 minutes a session.	____	____	____
· We incorporate activity in our family and work lives as much as possible.	____	____	____
· Our fitness plan includes stretching and rest periods.	____	____	____
· We choose exercise that is enjoyable.	____	____	____
· Our exercise plan includes activities that can be done individually or as a family.	____	____	____
· We use safety equipment, such as helmets and pads, when exercising.	____	____	____
· We limit use of television and other sedentary activities.	____	____	____

(continues)

EXHIBIT 8-5   Healthy Options Assessment *(continued)*

	Most of the time	Sometimes	Rarely
D. Rest and Relaxation			
· We honor each individual's sleep, rest, and relaxation patterns.	___	___	___
· Our children have regular bedtimes with calming bedtime rituals.	___	___	___
· Adults get 7 to 9 hours of sleep; children sleep 9 to 12 hours, depending on their age.	___	___	___
· We set aside time every week to relax and have fun as a family.	___	___	___
· Nap or quiet time is planned for those who choose or need it.	___	___	___
· We practice daily relaxation, such as breath work and meditation.	___	___	___
E. Financial Security/Household Responsibilities			
· Household chores and responsibilities are shared.	___	___	___
· Our income allows us to pay our bills on time.	___	___	___
· We have a long-range financial plan.	___	___	___
· Children have chores in addition to care of their possessions.	___	___	___
· We continually upgrade our work-related skills.	___	___	___
· The work we do honors us as individuals and as a family.	___	___	___
F. Family/Friends/Community			
· We have a nearby network of family and/or friends.	___	___	___
· We feel connected to our community.	___	___	___
· We participate in community groups and/or activities.	___	___	___
· Our community offers a positive quality of life for our family.	___	___	___
· We have regular get-togethers with family and/or friends.	___	___	___
· We are spiritually fulfilled through our religion and/or other spiritual activities.	___	___	___
G. Creative Expression			
· Family members are encouraged to use their individual talents.	___	___	___
· Family artwork is honored and displayed.	___	___	___
· Financial resources are allocated for lessons, equipment, or materials used in creative expression.	___	___	___
· All forms of creativity are valued, including culinary, financial, and athletic skills.	___	___	___
· We have rituals and celebrations that are unique to our family.	___	___	___

EXHIBIT 8-6   Issues for Discussion to Aid in Identifying Patterns Within the Family

· Identify those choices that promote balance and simplicity.

· Do you have a healthy amount of time together as a family? Do these occasions contribute to your well-being?

· Note how your choices support individual and family wellness.

· Determine whether your responses align with your family identity. Observe where they vary and explore the meaning of that variation.

· Ask yourself if your choices contribute to the health of your community.

· Which areas elicit an intuitive response of satisfaction, consternation, or anything in between? An intuitive response arises when you have observed something that has significance for you. Such an observation can indicate a pattern to continue because of its benefits. Conversely, your response may be rooted in a pattern that does not support health and warrants change.

---

who exhibit balanced living. When surveying the Healthy Options list, you will notice that following these guidelines requires commitment, communication, and coordination. Each family must decide which guidelines have meaning and which to disregard. Feel free to add any that will create an individualized profile of nourishing habits.

Patterns/Repatterning

After this exercise has been completed, it should be reviewed and put away for a few days. Resist the temptation to judge or analyze behaviors when you return to it. Survey the responses, looking for patterns that emerge. Exhibit 8-6 offers issues that can be reviewed to help identify patterns within the family.

It is useful for people to identify those healthy options areas that reflect their family's optimal functioning. This can be followed by noting those areas in which they would like to create change over the coming weeks or months. They should be guided in staying focused on keeping their goals reasonable and in alignment with their family identities. They may want to begin their change process with small goals that can be readily accomplished. After they have celebrated success and developed an atmosphere that fosters growth, they can select more challenging goals.

Goal Setting

There are steps families can follow to make concrete action plans that will help them to create what they want for the future (see Exhibit 8-7). This process is enriched by establish-

---

EXHIBIT 8-7   Goal-Setting Steps

1. Plan a time for the family to meet about a specific purpose, such as planning meals, choosing a pet, or selecting a vacation destination.

2. Set the goal. What is it you want to do? Does it fit within the picture of your family identity? Is it a reasonable goal given your resources of time, skills, and finances? Do you have a clear picture of what your goal will look and feel like once it has been reached?

3. Plan the process for reaching your objective. Design a long-term plan with steps that can be accomplished in two to four weeks. This will make your efforts seem more reasonable because your gains will be readily visible. Working on short-term steps allows room for course corrections as your project unfolds.

4. Set aside time to review and celebrate your successes. It makes it easier to focus on your next steps when you can look back and pat yourself on the back for a job well done. Reflection serves to remind the entire family that everyone is in this together, no matter what the individual roles and responsibilities are.

5. Review and revise goals as needed. Sometimes in the course of a project the goal changes. It may be altered enough to look like a whole new goal. It may no longer be relevant, being dropped entirely or reframed into a new goal. For instance, a family was in the process of planning to purchase a larger home. They explored their options and decided that, given low interest rates and love of their current home, it was better to build an addition than to purchase a new home.

6. Recognize goal attainment. This is an opportunity to review your change process and to identify alterations you will make in it when you establish goals for future projects. It also is a time to celebrate success in reaching desired outcomes.

---

ing equality: Each person has a chance to be heard, to state opinions, to offer suggestions, and to describe their role in family goal setting and goal attainment.

Changing habits and adopting new life patterns can often be accomplished through small shifts in behavior. For example, if people want to become more physically active, they can increase activity at work by going for a 10-minute walk rather than taking the usual coffee break.

KEY POINT

Adopting small actions that can be readily integrated into the daily routine increases the success of a plan.

These ideas are not new. Most people have heard them before, time and again. If behavior changes have been attempted in the past without success, perhaps there has been an intent to alter too much at once. Change takes time and a modest approach. Look for small, healthy changes that can be easily accomplished. Remember that habits are developed over time. Weeks or months of practice may be needed before positive effects of actions are noted.

REFLECTION

One action-oriented example of a healthy change involves your daily routine travel. Whether you travel by car, train, or bus, take three breaths when you arrive at your destination. The 15 or 20 seconds you invest in this routine will clear your mind and cleanse your body. Do you think you are worthy of this modest investment?

Holistic Parenting

Holistic parenting is based on mindfulness, kindness, respect, and reflection. Through the parent/child relationship, people learn more about themselves while learning about their child. They come to honor their individuality as much as you cherish their common traits. They learn to listen to their hearts, the wisdom centers that will guide them to parent in a way that is respectful and prepares their children and themselves for the future. They learn that discipline is another way of caring.

Parenting, once started in a holistic and loving way, lasts a lifetime. Parents become the family elders. As people age and grow in their parenting experiences, they will reflect more on their own lessons; they will see that their children also have lessons to learn through their own experiences. They will stand as guides and supporters, pointing the way and offering a heart and hand when the going is rough.

KEY POINT

The challenge of being a parent is to live our moments as fully as possible, charting our own courses as best we can, above all, nourishing our children, and in the process, growing ourselves. Our children and the journey itself provide us with endless opportunities in this regard.[3]

Topics that are discussed in this section will build on or reflect back to the exercises completed in the section about balancing family, work, and leisure. Through holistic awareness, people will develop a realization that there are many paths to follow when parenting a child. Although there are those who will suggest, prod, coerce, even mandate that people parent in a specific manner, ultimately, all parents are responsible to their own children and to themselves for the form their parenting will assume.

Holistic parenting is based on strength-oriented practice. It maintains a focus on personal competence while promoting positive traits and behaviors. The child is honored for whom he or she is and the attributes radiated as a unique person while being guided with clear, reasonable, and healthy expectations. This practice does not disregard less desired behaviors, actions, and words; rather, it educates on how to keep them in perspective. It is centered on the art of offering love and respect to a child while discussing challenging, frustrating, or painful situations.

KEY POINT

Mindful parenting involves being attentive, setting limits, having realistic expectations, and displaying fairness, consistency, and flexibility.

Holistic parenting can begin at any time; it is never too late. Humans are resilient and respond well to those who focus on their gifts and treat them with respect. When people parent from a heart center, they learn to apologize and to forgive with integrity and without the burden of guilt for either themselves or their children. This is a discipline; practice is necessary. Mindfully, they will do the best they can for today, and tomorrow they will arise and engage in their heart-centered practice again. At times, parents may feel that their parenting skills are developing more slowly than desired. Parents need to be encouraged to hold on to their intentions and to focus on their desires to have open, balanced relationships with their children.

Parenting Education from a Holistic Perspective

Parenting education, until recent years, has been primarily experiential. We learned about parenting as children from our parent' examples. We took those lessons and applied them to our children, making adjustments as each child grew or another came along. Anticipatory guidance, or what to expect in a child's development and how to prepare for and manage it, came primarily from well-meaning family and friends and information gathered during pediatrician visits. To add to our overall inexperience and confusion, points of view often varied, sometimes being contradictory.

Today there are parenting classes and support groups, books and videotapes, and community resources that provide specialized support and guidance for families. Many of these will ask parents to do the same thing: begin at the beginning. How do parents begin at the beginning when their child is 6 years old and they feel bogged down by patterns that are already established? Part of the beginning is going back to their own childhoods, to those earliest memories of their families. Parents can be guided to recall the faces and relationships, the good times and the bad. Questions can be asked: When were you happy? What made you run and hide? What do you do or say now that seems like a flashback from those long ago years?

Remembering those times and family patterns that brought them joy—or pain—can offer parents hints for what to do and avoid with their own children. Thinking back to those years can help people to become mindful parents. Moment by moment they will become aware of verbal habits, facial expressions, and mannerisms that have become embedded in their behavior patterns. The manner with which their children respond to their words and actions will give parents clues about which behaviors to continue and which to change. When parents release an unhealthy behavior from their past, they may be ending a family cycle that has been in place for generations. The legacy of their actions has the potential to extend past the lives of their children.

Another way to begin at the beginning is to study child development. This commitment to learn about development from the earliest moments of life in utero (in the uterus/womb) can help parents to understand children's behaviors. They will be less confused by the once friendly 7-month-old who now melts into tears as a reserved 10-month-old. They will understand why their practical 4-year-old has suddenly developed an intriguing relationship with an imaginary friend.

KEY POINT

There are predictable patterns of growth and development at various ages that parents need to understand.

Learning about development helps parents appreciate their children in relation to others of the same stage while gaining a sense of each child's temperament and talents. They learn to respect and have compassion for those parents whose child is intense, very shy, or has special needs. Sharing their joys and frustrations with other parents can help them to learn new techniques while guiding others by the example of their lessons. They come to realize they are not alone and that being with someone who listens fully while acknowledging their feelings is a precious gift.

When parents gain an understanding of child development they are better able to:

- Understand their children's words and actions
- Adjust their expectations to match their children's current level of ability and understanding
- Use behavioral guidance and discipline that is appropriate for a child's developmental level

- Anticipate what stages will come next and how to prepare for coming changes
- Provide a safe environment for a child
- Plan family activities that match a child's interests and abilities
- Offer foods that are interesting, safe, and nutritionally sound
- Help others to understand their children's individual talents, preferences, and challenges
- Understand the variations in development from one child to another and typical milestones (a milestone is the average age at which most children will develop a skill such as sitting up, talking, and walking)
- Know when they, their children, or their family need professional guidance and support regarding health, development, behaviors, or relationships
- Accept their children and others for the people they are and the individuals they are becoming
- Identify, acknowledge, and balance their personal needs with those of their children

---

REFLECTION (FOR PARENTS)

As you reflect on your own childhood experiences and what you have learned about "typical" (usual, average, expected) child development, pause to reflect on the thoughts that arise as you complete these statements:

- I became a parent because _____

_____

- I knew I wanted to be a parent when I _____

_____

- I hoped for a child who _____

_____

Sit with your responses, breathing gently into your heart. As you continue to breathe, release emotions that have manifested with your statements. Release any fear, sadness, and anger and allow yourself to be filled with peace, suspended in this eternal moment.

Hold that sense of peacefulness and proceed by completing these statements:

- As a parent I wish I could _____

_____

(continues)

REFLECTION (FOR PARENTS) *(continued)*

· The greatest gift I have given my child is _____

_____

· The greatest gift my child has given me is _____

_____

· The best advice I could give a new parent is _____

_____

· The person who is most supportive of me as a parent is _____

_____

· This person shows their support by _____

_____

Put your responses aside and breathe quietly for a few minutes. Review your statements without judgment. As you reflect on your statements, consider the following:

· Those that are strength-based, containing words that are positive, offering affirmation and a feeling of hope. Note where there are patterns of similarity or contradiction.
· Those statements that surprise you
· Those that bring up emotions: your joy, sadness, and anger

Write a page about what you have learned about how your original desires and expectations of parenting differ from your present reality. Define steps you can take to become a more effective parent over the coming year. Use your affirmative statements as the building blocks for what you want to accomplish. For instance, you could say, "I will use supportive listening and open dialogue to guide my child in seeking new solutions for problems at school."

Seeking Guidance

Disruption may signify that professional guidance is needed to help resolve a situation. That support could be available from a healthcare provider, a rabbi or minister, or a counselor. Today, there are numerous support groups and therapies, both traditional and complementary, for families who are seeking wisdom and solace.

Mutual trust and respect are two of the cornerstones on which a therapeutic relationship is based. People need to give themselves permission to search for the right match for their family. They should talk with the professional person about their beliefs and values, and the hopes they have for their parent/child relationship. They can then invite that person to partner with them as their parenting develops and as their children grow in life awareness.

Parents need to take time to center and find renewal in personally satisfying ways. When they feel whole and refreshed they have greater resources to bring to their relationships with their children. The children, in turn, will learn from their parents' example that personal time is important for maintaining health and balance. Parents need to encourage their children to find their own methods for relaxing and attaining personal fulfillment.

Family Comes Full Cycle

Our days go from dawn to dusk; our years flow from spring through winter. Thus it is with our lives and those of our family members.

We have touched on survival, balance, and each family's unique qualities. A person's individuality is embraced in the family's inherent rhythms and cycles. By pausing to recall past and plan for the future, a person becomes more keenly aware of those patterns.

Summary

Families come in a variety of forms, including blended, single-parent, one child, multiple children, same-gender partner, grandparents raising grandchildren, younger parents, older parents, and couples without children. There are some basic assumptions when working with families that can guide a professional's actions. Each family is unique, influences and is influenced by its community and culture, shares many things in common with other families, deserves respect and opportunities for success, and has responsibility to respect and care for its members while accepting the individuality of its members. Each family has a unique body, mind, and spirit.

The Healthy Options Assessment offered in this chapter can be useful in guiding families in the discussion of their patterns in regard to food, communication, displays of affection, physical activity, rest and relaxation, financial security, household responsibilities, family, friends, community, and creative expression. From this, plans can be made for repatterning.

Parenting should be viewed as a holistic process. It is based on mindfulness, kindness, and reflection. It is a strength-oriented practice. With reflection, knowledge, and practice, parenting patterns can improve.

References

1. Merriam Webster Online Dictionary. Accessed January 1, 2008 from http://www.m-w.com/dictionary/leisure
2. Kabat Zinn, M., & Kabat Zinn, J. (2000). *Everyday Blessings*. New York: Hyperion, p. 24.
3. Kabat Zinn, M., & Kabat Zinn, J. (2000). *Everyday Blessings*. New York: Hyperion, p. 3.

Suggested Reading

Bolles, R. N. (2007). *What Color Is Your Parachute? 2008*. Berkeley, CA: Ten Speed Press.
Covey, S. (1999). *The Seven Habits of Highly Effective Families*. New York: St. Martin's Griffin.

Fosarelli, P. D. (2006). *Ages, Stages, and Phases: from Infancy to Adolescence: Integrating Physical, Social, Emotional, Intellectual, and Spiritual Development*. Liguori, MO: Liguori Press.

Gluck, B. R., & Rosenfeld, J. (2005). *How to Survive Your Teenager: By Hundreds of Still-Sane Parents Who Did and Some Things to Avoid, From a Few Whose Kids Drove Them Nuts*. Atlanta, GA: Hundreds of Heads Books.

Goldberg, H., & Goldberg, I. (2007). *Family Therapy: An Overview*. New York: Brooks Cole.

St. James, E. (2000). *Simplify Your Life with Kids*. Kansas City: Andrews McMeel Publishing.

Schor, E. L. (ed.). (1999). *Caring for Your School Age Child*. New York: Bantam Books.

Shelov, S. (ed.). (2004). *Caring for Your Baby and Young Child*, revised edition. New York: Bantam Books.

Wright, H. N. (2004). *How to Talk So Your Kids Will Listen*. Ventura, CA: Regla Books.

Chapter 9

The Spiritual Connection

OBJECTIVES

This chapter should enable you to

· Describe the differences between spirituality and religion

· Describe the process of letting go of preconceived notions

· List two elements of spiritual preparation

· Discuss the healing value of service to others

In recent years, there has been considerable emphasis on eating a nutritious diet, exercising regularly, and taking other actions to a healthy lifestyle. Many consumers have responded by adopting positive practices and taking an active interest in their health. Even conventional medicine has slowly, yet progressively, incorporated some common sense lifestyle suggestions into patient care.

Health, however, is influenced by more than just the maintenance of the body. From a holistic perspective, the individual is comprised of body, mind, and spirit. Each of these components impacts the others and influences health.

Increasingly, research is shedding light on the relationship between spirituality and health. People who are spiritually fulfilled and engage in regular spiritual practices tend to enjoy higher health states than those who do not. On the other hand, persons with ideal physical bodies who are spiritually empty or distressed fall short of meeting an optimal health status.

KEY POINT

Spirituality is not synonymous with religion.

Spirituality and Religion

Looking past the worship practices and belief systems of organized religion, you can move into an integrated dimension of wholeness known as spirituality. Being essential to life, spirituality reflects the common threads that flow through all religions and belief systems. Spirituality embraces all aspects of every living thing: the mind, the body, and the spirit. From this larger perspective in consciousness, you embrace life and life's issues from a place of collective being and knowing. This is different from the choices involved in practicing a religion.

REFLECTION

How are spirituality and religion viewed and expressed differently in your life?

Spirituality is simply being. Religion is like following a map that was charted to keep people on a predetermined single path toward a destination. Spirituality is similar to sitting on top of a mountain where insight is gained from a larger viewpoint, which draws one to the best path. As perspective widens from religion to spirituality, people begin to realize the unity and connectedness of all things. This innate state of being is essential to life. It is that place that enables people to know their authentic selves. Spirituality does not negate religion; rather, it shows where the commonalities or universal truths among all beliefs are founded.

When comparing spirituality and religion, some interesting differences can be noted. Words defining religion relate to belief systems and practices of worship that can vary from culture to culture. Words used to define spirituality have a wider universal expression that goes beyond religion and opens you to a greater awareness of one's true being (see Exhibit 9-1).

Spirituality as a Broader Perspective

From a broader perspective of spirituality, commonalities among all religions and beliefs can be seen. There is a unifying force, a power, a presence, an essence to life that is greater than the individual, yet encompasses all human beings and all living things.

KEY POINT

That which represents the spiritual dimension is represented by many names and ideas, such as God, Jesus Christ, Chi, Allah, Great Spirit, Infinite Intelligence, Unconditional Love, Goddess, Universal Life Force, Intuition, Higher Power, and, most simply, from India, The Energy.

Spirituality impacts everything people say, think, and do. This ornate tapestry of interconnectedness expands from the individual to other people, places, and things. Seeing a beautiful picture or experiencing great music can fill one with love and rapture of emotions.

Exhibit 9-1	Common Words Associated with Spirituality and Religion
Spirituality	**Religion**
Ethereal	Belief
Airy	Creed
Holy	Faith
Higher Power	Church
Sacred	Cult
Essence	Sect
Transcendence	Theology
Being	Doctrine

Still expanding in unity and connectedness, the connection with nature, the planet, and the universe is also realized. One can become lost in a beautiful sunset, enjoying and connecting with it so much that for a few moments the sunset is all that there is. This connectedness also means experiencing pain and hurt, as well as beauty and inspiration. Pictures of a war-torn country can cause people to feel the pain, sorrow, and hardship of its victims.

From this place of seeing and experiencing, people begin to comprehend on a deeper level, the spiritual level. Seeing that what happens to the one affects everything and what happens to everything affects the one. This often results in a sense of awe or inspiration as people discover this Creative Force/God in everything.

Planetary Connectedness

In this place of awareness and connectedness, many people are discovering a deep reverence for the planet. There is an awareness that the abuse of the planet not only affects the earth, but each of its inhabitants. The individual affects the planet and the planet affects the individual. The individual's health affects the community and the community's health affects an individual's health. The individual, the community, the nation, and the world are all connected.

Being, Knowing, and Doing

In considering spirituality, *being, knowing*, and *doing* take on new meanings. People become more aware of their inner selves and begin to intuitively sense what to do and how to do it. They begin to feel more comfortable acting on these feelings. Herein lies the essence of the spiritual connection and the beginning of healing.

Being is the art, the awareness of the here and now, or the present. There are no thoughts—only stillness—and with stillness comes awareness through all the senses. The mind becomes quiet and just is. This stillness heightens the awareness of each of the senses even more. This place of stillness with self, others, and the environment enables one to experience the moment on a deeper level. It is as though the body is responding to observations from all of the senses. This state is often referred to as being centered or balanced; yet, it is more.

REFLECTION

Experience Being:

> Take a deep breath and gently release it.
>
> Feel how the mind releases with the body.
>
> Take another deep breath and another.
>
> Notice how each breath permits the body and mind to relax even further
>
> Now take a breath and as you exhale, linger in the exhalation.

From this larger place of being, people begin to express with greater awareness, peace, and connectedness rather than from desires, self-centeredness, or envy. It is in this place of awareness and peace that healing takes place.

Knowing comes from being open to all things, not just the ones we have stored in our memory. There is a deep inner sense of awareness of things and their interactions and effects. This knowing is accompanied with a feeling of openness or lightness in the entire body.

REFLECTION

Experience Knowing:

> Close your eyes.
>
> Take some slow, deep breaths with gentle exhalations.
>
> Scan your body for any tight places.
>
> Gently breathe into the tight areas.
>
> Remain in this easy breathing.
>
> Notice that your body is becoming lighter and lighter.
>
> Feel the freedom and lightness with each breath.
>
> Feel the gentle lightness—almost tingling.
>
> Continue with this breathing.
>
> Stay in this place of freedom and healing as long as you desire.

Often people come to recognize that they reach a place of clarity and right thought when the knowing and the light feeling come at the same time. It is like the tingling or lightness is validating or confirming the clarity of the knowing. This is a natural intelligence unrelated to physical memory. This natural intelligence is intuition, one's energy talking. It lets people know what they need to be doing. It tells them what is and is not supportive, what opens or constricts them, and what makes them feel heavy or light. Knowing comes with sensing and feeling this natural intelligence.

From this inner place of being and knowing emerges doing. This outward expression is spirituality made visible. Doing starts with individuals taking care of themselves in healthy, loving, life-giving ways. Honoring knowing and being is sometimes a challenge, especially when being and knowing conflict with expectations imposed by self or others.

Learning from Relationships

The ability for people to experience and express themselves from a wider consciousness is an evolving process. Relationships are the school for this growth in spirituality. People are in a relationship with everything in their lives . . . other people, places, things, themselves, and their Higher Powers. All desires for fame, fortune, and to get ahead are transient happiness as they are nonrelational. Ultimately, the nonrelational aspects of life increase the hunger for the real relationship, the inner connection, the spiritual connection with a power greater than self.

Some people may spend considerable time trying to fix things on the outside when their need is to respond to their deepest calling. They may want to change jobs, improve their image, live in an upscale community, or lose weight. The changing and fixing of these outer things brings some satisfaction for a brief period, but then the novelty wears off and they must be attended to once again. Striving for satisfaction through outer means is indicative of a need for a deeper inner relationship with being.

The deepest calling, the deepest yearning, is to know and remember one's connectedness and oneness to something greater than oneself. As people begin to realize the power and peace of this unity, this oneness in their lives, they begin to desire and experience connectedness more and more. They begin to realize that this connectedness is almost magical and most certainly sacred. Seeking this Inner Light or Higher Power, individuals find that the unity that feeds the spirit is more important than their physical pleasures or dreams of wealth and prestige. They are able to let go of having to create images and control others and events, and, as they let go, their lives and health begin to change.

KEY POINT

Releasing all need for control, one can move with love, joy, and clarity in the moment.

Abundance is a simple yet profound truth of the universe. When people want and move into the eternal more than the ephemeral, they begin to experience a peace that surpasses all understanding. They discover the unconditional love that sees beyond all outward appearances and behaviors. They feel the inner joy that is always there, independent of what is happening in their lives.

How people deal with outer relationships reflects their state of consciousness and inner awareness of who they really are. The emotional personality, that constricted ego place in consciousness, is like blinders on a horse that keep it looking and moving only in one direction while ignoring many of the things nearby. Living without blinders allows people to experience the expansive spiritual place and see the joy and beauty of everything around them. Spirituality assists in examining emotions, behaviors, and attitudes. Without the blinders, individuals can see more clearly the limitations that constrain them in self-serving, destructive thinking. The individual can be his or her own best teacher. By observing how they respond to others and their deeper motivations, people can begin to understand the purposes behind their actions. This insight can guide them in discovering the blocks and hindrances to healthy, joyous relationships. They begin to identify the ideas that keep them locked in limitation, disease, and imbalance.

KEY POINT

Native Americans instruct their youth to look beyond to discover truth. After that truth has been discovered, one looks beyond, again and again until one has reached the essence of universal truth.

Individuals' relationships with others demonstrate the limitations that they hold in their minds. Their judgments and pronouncements only lead to a frustrating cycle of trying to fix someone else. Rather than thinking and acting in a limiting and tightening manner, they need to loosen up and allow themselves to be open, accepting, and free. When they release the preconceived notions of how things should work or how others should act, life begins to flow easily. The mind and body respond by being in balance; this is health.

REFLECTION

Experience Letting Go:

Consider a recent situation that caused you to become unsettled.

Look at the reason for the emotion.

Now look beyond that reason to the underlying reason.

Keep looking beyond to the next reason and the next until you reach the core reason and can go no further.

Take slow deep breaths and gently release them.

Remain in this place of peace and ease as long as you like.

Being Honest

Being honest with oneself is an important part of healthy living. Honestly going within may reveal things that people may not feel comfortable discovering, but this process could help them to discover the blinders and falsehoods that have been accepted as being real. Take this example:

A college administrator was sitting at her desk perplexed at the response she was receiving from her faculty regarding the proposed curriculum changes. She kept attempting to figure out how to present the curriculum so that the changes would be accepted. In her silence and quiet breathing, she realized that she was manipulating the faculty to do things her way, rather than being open to their recommendations for changes. It felt awful to see herself in the role of a manipulator when she had thought of herself as an empowering leader. Releasing this, she stayed with her breathing and went deeper. She realized that she needed to present the facts as clearly as possible and allow the faculty to make decisions. The administrator let go of any need to have the curriculum changes fit her preconceived idea and opened herself to the faculty's suggestions. The faculty moved together and improved the curriculum beyond everyone's expectations.

When issues are seen for what they really are, people are in a better position to release them. These issues no longer have control and people can move deeper into a place of clarity, healing, and being.

There is a saying that insanity is doing the same thing and expecting different results. Stopping the insanity is paramount to being honest. If a person's joints are stiff each morning after drinking wine the previous evening, why does he or she keep drinking the wine and expecting different results? If life is not working, if a person is not healthy and not moving in a healthy direction, it is time to do something different. Often, insights and guidance provided by a healthcare professional can help individuals clarify unhealthy habits and initiate actions to change them.

Gratitude

Gratitude comes in continually larger and larger doses as one takes the time to go within and be quiet. The vicious cycles of anger, fear, and resentment are replaced with love, knowing, being, and increasing awareness. Spirituality soon permeates every part of life, giving guidance, comfort, healing, purpose, and direction. The body and mind are taken to new levels of connectedness, and a person is able to see the unity and beauty in everything.

KEY POINT

As spiritual awareness is heightened, a person begins to feel thankful for the ordinary—a new day, the ability to get out of bed independently, a job that can provide the means to keep a roof over one's head and food in one's stomach, the support of loved ones. These aspects of everyday life that often are taken for granted can, instead, be appreciated as special gifts.

Prayer is an expression of gratitude. People can express appreciation that they are being protected and blessed as they face that which is before them and also give thanks for the protection and blessings that have been experienced. Prayers of thanksgiving reflect a connection with a higher power and contribute to feelings of abundance.

Forgiveness

Virtually all human beings have had the experience of someone hurting or wronging them in some manner. Sometimes the offense was so severe and the subsequent pain so strong that it is difficult to accept an apology and forgive the person. Nevertheless, there are other times when the offending individual fails to apologize or ask for forgiveness.

Forgiveness is not only the process of forgiving those who come to you asking for forgiveness but also offering forgiveness without being asked. It may seem difficult to consider forgiving a person who has done something bad to you or hurt you when that individual has not even apologized or sought forgiveness. Nevertheless, by not forgiving, you keep the wound of pain open and cause yourself continued suffering.

Forgiveness is an act that yields more benefit for you than for the one forgiven. It is liberating and a necessary step to healing from the incident. Also, the stress relieved through the act of forgiveness offers multiple health benefits, including reducing depression and anxiety, improving heart rate and blood pressure.[1-3]

Forgiveness does not imply that the act was condoned or excused but, rather, that you have made the decision to not allow the emotional cloud of unforgiveness to hang over you and continue to control you. You may not forget the incident, but you do not have to be imprisoned by the emotions it generates, such as anger, bitterness, and resentment.

KEY POINT

When moving toward the process of forgiveness, it is useful to ask yourself these questions:

·   What burden am I carrying by not releasing the feelings associated with the incident?
·   Is it worth occupying my mind and spirit with the negative feelings arising from continuing to be angry or resentful about the incident rather than freeing that space for positive feelings?
·   Have I ever wronged someone and been given the gift of forgiveness?
·   What example do I want to set for others?

Spirituality as Lived Experience

Spirituality is a daily experience highlighted with some peak experiences. Within the unity and connectedness, a sense of order and natural balance in life and in the world exists. One discovers that there is no single path to spirituality, no road map. Spirituality simply *is*. This is a lived experience and a moment-by-moment awakening and discovering of one's true being. Things that used to baffle a person in the past become understood and manageable. Problems are viewed as opportunities to learn and grow. Unhealthy habits begin to melt away. An individual begins to respond from a different place in consciousness.

REFLECTION

You have probably heard of situations in which people risked their lives to help others in emergency situations. They immediately responded and did what was necessary at the time without consideration of the personal risks and dangers. Can you think of a time when you or someone close to you took this type of risk?

When guided by spirit, there is no fear but rather, being, knowing, and doing. Fear enters when the mind leads. Being is a place of no fear—no peripheral thoughts or emotions—just total presence in the moment. Fear comes from one's memory of personal experiences or what others have led him or her to fear (e.g., warnings from persons in authority or situations described in the media). The memory collects everything that is happening in the environment whether a person is aware of it or not. This collection of memory is what is used as a standard against which current situations are measured. This memory, although helpful at times, can keep a person locked into certain beliefs, ideas, and concepts.

Resisting the temptation to be limited by the memories that have guided their actions in the past, people can face the present without fear. They will learn to trust that they will not be harmed or overwhelmed, which can help them to discover happiness, joy, and spontaneity unlike anything experienced before.

REFLECTION

During the day, observe your thoughts when something unexpected happens. Do you respond with anxiety and fear or with confidence that you will be able to handle the situation?

Moving to Solutions

Throughout life people experience many challenges in their relationships, health, work, and family lives. When challenges continue beyond what people feel is reasonable they may begin to get concerned, worried, and fearful. Prayers do not seem to be answered, and they may begin to question, usually silently, whether there really is a God, an infinite intelligence. At these times, it feels as if they will never be free of the challenge. These experiences offer an opportunity to either be part of the solution or part of the problem. Moving to solutions expands and opens people to positive ideas, thoughts, and a way through the situation, whereas remaining in the problem keeps them locked in the role of victim. Helping people to move to solutions empowers them to act, change, and discover the path to managing the situation effectively.

Complaining is an example of an activity that causes people to remain in their problems. For example, a person may telephone several friends complaining about a situation, repeating the same story each time. She may be so consumed with complaining that she does not take the time to reflect and consider possibilities for changing the situation, somewhat like a person who complains about being hot and thirsty but who fails to take a drink of water! It is when the person is willing to let go of the problem that she can move into the solution.

When people have a challenge or a health problem in their lives, they need to take the time to be quiet and still and go within. In this place of stillness, there is no talking, just quiet. Focusing on their breathing they become peaceful and let go of the fear, the judgments, the blame, and all of the defenses that may contribute to this challenge.

REFLECTION

Moving to Solutions:

Close your eyes and begin to take long, slow breaths.

Gently allow the exhalations to become longer than the inhalations.

Focus on your breathing. If necessary say, "Breathe in, breathe out."

Feel the tension, fear, judgments, and blame leaving.

Accept and know that peace and harmony are filling you.

Remain in this place of peace until you naturally come back.

Simply feeling the experience of peace and harmony is a very powerful type of prayer, a very powerful healing process. It is this feeling of peace that works the magic.

KEY POINT

Life is about expanding. People become small when they remain in the problem. As they become still and peaceful, inner knowing emerges, and they become whole again. Wholeness begins in thought and then is expressed in the physical.

Spiritual Preparation for Health and Healing

Increasing time in conscious connection and stillness brings people into a place of expanding peace, love, and healing. They begin to feel extremely positive and safe, as though nothing can go wrong; however, their comfort can cause them to be surprised and taken off guard when difficulties arise.

Pilots take time before each flight to do a preflight check of the craft and its instrumentation. They know that this preparation helps to ensure a smooth flight because problems are handled before the plane leaves the ground. Like the pilot, people can spare themselves some problems and function more smoothly by starting each day with a check of their minds, bodies, and spirits. A daily time of quiet reflection can clarify the challenges that are present and assist in resolving issues. This time of daily reflection—sometimes called prayer, personal private time, getting quiet, meditation—is a time of being reflective and honest with the self. It gives one the opportunity to work on unresolved emotional issues. When people begin to see the areas of life that are being threatened, then they are able to determine how these threats repeatedly appear in different forms. After they identify the blocks to health, peace, and love, they can turn these blocks over to a Higher Power and continue with living and being. They are taking action to control their threats rather than be controlled by them.

> **REFLECTION**
>
> **Identifying Patterns:**
>
> With paper and pencil in hand, find a quiet place.
>
> Review your day.
>
> Select a current issue or problem.
>
> In two or three words, state why it is a problem.
>
> Ask what area or areas of your life are being threatened: personal relations, sexual relations, financial security, emotional security, and self-esteem.
>
> Select another issue, and repeat the process.
>
> Continue repeating the process until all of the day's issues have been identified.
>
> Look for similarities in causes among the issues. These are the patterns that restrict your life.

Imagine that you have a very special friend whom you hold in great esteem. This wonderful and fantastic friend takes care of your requests. After you tell this friend about whatever areas of your life are being threatened, you immediately feel secure, light, and free. Wouldn't it be great to have a friend like this? People do. This friend goes by many names: **God, Jesus Christ, Higher Power, Infinite Intelligence, the Absolute,** or **Creator**.

The second part of spiritual preparation is having faith that everything is being taken care of and that there is nothing more that one needs to do. When you instruct the computer with a series of commands, you often get a "please wait" comment on the screen while the computer is working on the instructions. Likewise, when things are turned over to God or a Higher Power, people often get a "please wait" message, although this response may not be communicated as obviously as the message on a computer screen. Individuals must go about their lives and trust that the Higher Power is in charge and taking care of everything. When worry is released to a Higher Power, it is no longer necessary to think or obsess over it. This also means that not only is the outcome out of one's control but that it also may not be what one envisioned. Sometimes what we want is not what we really need.

Service as Healing

In the process of healing people can become quite absorbed in changing the effects or symptoms in their lives. It soon becomes clear that as long as they stay focused on themselves they will not be fully connected to the whole. In truth, they are part of everything: the planet, the universe, and the situations happening around them. All of these affect reality. When people personalize illness, it keeps them separated from the whole; they can blame others, their situations, and themselves. When they move illness from a personal to a larger perspective, their primary consciousness is altered—a change from the blaming, self-serving ego into the expanded awareness of the unity, and connectedness of all things.

From this larger perspective, people can begin to realize that a critical part of healing is being of service to others. As long as they are focused on themselves, people do not completely heal. They need to discover that to receive they must give; to be loved, they must be loving, and to heal, they must be healing to others. There can be no receiving without giving.

KEY POINT

The universal law of giving and receiving is interactive and circular: One cannot occur without the other.

Being of service comes in all shapes and forms—offering a glass of water to a thirsty traveler, paying the difference at the cash register for some one who is short of cash, calling someone who is feeling isolated and down, washing a daughter's new dress by hand, volunteering to clean the gutters of a neighbor's home. Service without motive creates an atmosphere of love and joy. The only reason for doing is the pure act of love and connectedness. In order to be healed one must be in the place of service to others, to administer to others without any motive except to give.

Health Benefits of Faith

Faith has been accepted and recognized as very powerful through the ages. This includes faith in oneself, in what one is doing, in friends, and in God. Faith is much more than just the religious experience of faith, although the highest expression of faith is in the spiritual attitude.

Frequently, the main element lacking in prayer life and daily life is faith. People pray, turn things over to a Higher Power, and then dig them up to see if they have sprouted or taken root.

REFLECTION

How often do you ask for assistance and then take your troubles back and worry about them, rather than trusting that help will be provided?

Faith establishes a rapport with the infinite. There is the realization that whatever is happening, a Higher Power is in complete charge. Everything is moving in divine concert for the highest and best. Faith opens people not only to healing, but to all the activities that support that healing process—diet, exercise, environment, and thinking patterns.

Faith means a conviction that one can trust that there is a purpose for everything and that occurrences will ultimately yield a greater good. People must nurture faith and release thoughts that would in any way weaken this conviction. The attitudes of belief, acceptance, and trust build and nourish faith. Any thoughts that threaten or weaken any of these attitudes, even in the slightest, also weaken faith. When thinking is in line, then the healing process is accelerated.

Attention, Attitudes, and Healing

Attention, attitudes, and healing are invisible, yet their effects are constantly producing visible forms in life. If this thought life is not aligned and in balance, there will be painful consequences. Where individuals place their attention is what they bring into their lives. When they focus on problems, they potentially are inviting more problems. By focusing on pain, they experience more pain; by focusing on the relief of the pain, they experience comfort.

REFLECTION

Where Is Your Attention?

Wait until you are thirsty.

Fill a glass half full with water.

Observe your thoughts.

Are you seeing the glass half empty or half full?

Are you thinking about how good the water will taste or that it won't be enough?

Are you thinking about how your thirst will be quenched or that you will still be thirsty?

Where is your attention?

Simply observing breathing will reveal much about how individuals are responding to a situation. When people become constricted in their thinking or are becoming fearful about something, their breathing becomes shallow. People need to be taught that when this change in breathing is observed, they need to breathe deeply and remind themselves that their Higher Power is in charge, not the fear or the doubts of the life situation.

People are living an endless and ever-expanding experience. Only by expanding the mind and spirit can one evolve, grow, and heal. When bound by the past with all its constrictions and predetermined ways to do things, people are contracting. When they breathe deeply and allow themselves to move past this, they expand consciousness and enter into new understandings of unity and connectedness with a Higher Power.

People have the opportunity to begin life anew—to have the opportunity to set into motion the deeper positive attitudes that heal. They can either stay where they are and repeat their mistakes of the past in different forms, or they can change their attitudes and the attention of their thoughts. Through attention and the observation of their thoughts, they come into alignment with awareness and its health and healing properties. They become where they place their attention.

REFLECTION

Read this story, and consider whether you have witnessed similar experiences in your life. Think about what a health professional could do to lead more people to behave like Beth.

There were three women who all lived in the same town; they all had the same type of breast cancer in the same location at the same time. They all went to the same doctor. When Sally heard the diagnosis, she cried and felt that her life had ended. She could think of nothing else but the dreaded course of the disease and how she was going to die. She was dead within 6 months. June received the news with mixed emotions and vacillated between being dreadfully depressed and feeling rather well about the prognosis and treatment. She had treatments on and off for 3 years, gradually going downhill and finally dying. Beth was shocked to hear the news of her breast cancer and went home and shared it with her husband. She spent time getting quiet, reading about the symptoms, and finding the treatment that felt the best for her. She discovered tapes, books, and friends that talked and worked in positive thinking. Her attention was on healing—herself, her family, and others. Twenty years later she is doing well, still focusing on healing—herself, her family and others.

When attention is coupled with an attitude of healing, movement can begin toward new solutions. People will begin to feel and know that healing is taking place in every aspect of their lives. Every time they realize they strayed from this place of high watch they can return. The art of realization is enough to take them out of the negative thoughts. It is as though they have become the watcher of their thoughts rather than being their thoughts. They can move back into the center of all life and allow peace to substitute for judgment, anger, and impatience. Being here in the present moment is the place of peace, healing, truth, and oneness with the Infinite.

KEY POINT

Be here NOW.

The Spiritual Connection

We came from a perfect creator. Our essence is whole, perfect, and complete. We are our creator in microcosm. Health, healing, and balance are already present.

The task of every person is to know wholeness, health, perfection, and completeness in his or her mind and heart right now; to recognize his or her perfection as a spiritual being. There should be no doubts, no disbeliefs, no maybes—simply assurance in knowing. Any beliefs that do not support this must be released. As the mind becomes cleared from doubt and limitation, one is able to discover radiant health and healing.

Summary

Although spirituality is a thread within religion, it is a broader concept than religion. It entails the relationship with a higher power that can be identified by various names by different people. It is important to health and healing for individuals to get in touch with their spirituality. This can be facilitated by establishing a daily quiet time for reflection, letting go of preconceived notions of how things should go and how people should act, turning things over to a Higher Power, and serving others.

References

1. Lansky, M. R. (2007). Unbearable shame, splitting, and forgiveness in the resolution of vengefulness. *Journal of the American Psychoanalytical Association, 55*(2):571–593.
2. Ufema, J. (2007). The power of forgiveness. *Nursing, 37*(12):28.
3. Mayo Clinic. (2008). Finding forgiveness: a path to better well-being. *Mayo Clinic Womens Healthsource, 12*(1):7.

Suggested Reading

Anderson, M., & Burggraf, V. (2008). Passing the torch: transcendence. *Geriatric Nursing, 28*(1):37–38.

Autry, J. A. (2002). *The Spirit of Retirement. Creating A Life of Meaning and Personal Growth.* New York: Prima Press.

Barnum, B. S. (2006). *Spirituality in Nursing* (2nd ed.). New York: Springer Publishing Company.

Craig, C., Weinert, C., Walton, J., & Derwinski-Robinson, B. (2006). Spirituality, chronic illness, and rural life. *Journal of Holistic Nursing, 24*(1):27–35.

Conway, J. (1997). *Men in Midlife Crisis.* Colorado Springs, CO: Chariot Victor Publications.

Dass, R. (2002). *One-Liners: A Mini Manual for a Spiritual Life.* New York: Bell Tower.

Dean, A. (1997). *Growing Older, Growing Better: Daily Meditations for Celebrating Aging.* Carlsbad, CA: Hay House.

Dossey, L. (1997). *Prayer Is Good Medicine.* New York: HarperCollins.

Dossey, L. (1999). *Reinventing Medicine: Beyond Mind–Body to a New Era of Healing.* San Francisco: Harper.

Dossey, L. (2003). *Healing the Body: Medicine and the Infinite Reach of the Mind.* London: Random House.

Hillman, J. (1999). *The Force of Character and the Lasting Life.* New York: Random House.

Kellemen, R. W., & Edwards, K. A. (2007). *Beyond Suffering: Embracing the Legacy of African American Soul Care and Spiritual Direction.* Grand Rapids, MI: Baker Books.

Kimble, M. A., McFadden, S. H., Ellor, J. W., & Seeber, J. J. (eds.). (2004). *Aging, Spirituality, and Religion.* Minneapolis: Fortress Press.

Kirkland, K. H., & McIlveen, H. (2000). *Full Circle: Spiritual Therapy for the Elderly.* Binghamton, NY: Haworth Press.

Koenig, H. G. (1994). *Aging and God. Spiritual Pathways to Mental Health in Midlife and Later Years.* New York: Haworth Pastoral Press.

Larson, D. B., Sawyers, J. P., & McCullough, M. E. (eds.) (1998). *Scientific Research on Spirituality and Health: A Consensus Report.* Rockville, MD: National Institute for Healthcare Research.

Lindberg, D. A. (2005). Integrative review of research related to meditation, spirituality, and the elderly. *Geriatric Nursing, 26*(6):372–327.

Mcsherry, W. (2006). *Making sense of spirituality in nursing and health care* (2nd ed.). Philadelphia: Jessica Kingley Publishers.

Myss, C. (1996). *Anatomy of the Spirit.* New York: Three Rivers Press.

O'Brien, M. E. (2007). *Spirituality in Nursing: Standing on Holy Ground* (3rd ed.). Sudbury, MA: Jones and Bartlett.

Pargament, K. I. (2001). *The Psychology of Religion and Coping.* New York: Guilford Press.

Rice, R. (1999). A little art in home care: Poetry and storytelling for the soul. *Geriatric Nursing, 20*(3):165–166.

Rybarczyk, B., & Bellg, A. (1997). *Listening to Life Stories.* New York: Springer.

Schweitzer, R., Norberg, M., & Larson, L. (2002). The parish nurse coordinator: a bridge to spiritual health care leadership for the future. *Journal of Holistic Nursing, 20*:212–231.

Shelly, J. A., & Miller, A. B. (1999). *Called to Care: A Christian Theology of Nursing.* Downers Grove, IL: InterVarsity Press.

Stanley, C. (1997). *The Blessings of Brokenness.* Grand Rapids, MI: Zondervan Publishing House.

VandeCreek, L. (1998). *Scientific and Pastoral Perspectives on Intercessory Prayer.* New York: Harrington Park Press.

Wallace, S. (2000). Rx RN: a spiritual approach to aging. *Alternative and Complementary Therapies, 6*(1):47–48.

Wilt, D. L., & Smucker, C. J. (2001). *Nursing the Spirit.* Washington, DC: American Nurses Publishing.

Wimberly, A. S. (1997). *Honoring African American Elders: A Ministry in the Soul Community.* San Francisco: Jossey-Bass.

Chapter 10

Balancing Work and Life

OBJECTIVES

This chapter should enable you to

- Define *work*
- List three purposes of work
- Describe at least eight characteristics of a positive work attitude
- List three negative work experiences
- Describe at least three measures to convert negative work experiences into positive work experiences

"Good living and good work go together. Life and livelihood ought not to be separated but to flow from the same source, which is Spirit, for both life and livelihood are about Spirit."[1] Life and work are about living with meaning, intention, joy, and a sense of contributing to the order and harmony of the family, community, and the universe.

Various Meanings of Work

Work generally is defined as an effort directed to produce or accomplish something. We work to provide ourselves with goods and services needed for life. Work is simply part of life; however, work is far from a simple term.

Work has different meanings for different people, often as a result of their experiences with work. Some people say they are lucky because work does not feel like work to them. They claim their work is enjoyable and satisfying regardless of the monetary reward. One wonders why these people are reluctant to identify work as work. What does the word *work* mean to these people? Why do they associate the term *work* with something undesirable?

Others connect work only with drudgery, toil, travail, and slavery. They consider work as something to be avoided as much as possible. They may say, "If I could only win the sweepstakes, I would never work again." One wonders if they would really be satisfied to live the rest of their lives in total leisure. Is it really work they abhor or the work in which they are currently engaged?

Many people associate work with earning money and consider any activity for which they receive pay work. Nevertheless, not all work is paid work. Those who devote their time to rearing children and caring for sick or disabled loved ones in their homes, for example, are often considered unemployed, even though they are surely working. As caretakers they use their talents to provide service to others and may even be aware of the purposes of their service in the universe. Their work is sometimes fascinating, delightful, rewarding, and joyful, but at times it is also demanding, distressing, frustrating, sad, mysterious, and even frightening. Although caretaking may not be acknowledged as work, most people do understand that it is important and contributes to the good of society.

REFLECTION

What does work mean to you? What has influenced your thoughts about what constitutes work?

Work contributes to self-development, thereby serving a purpose greater than the collection of a paycheck or production of goods and services. Work causes most people to feel productive, satisfied, and worthwhile; therefore, the need to work remains even when sufficient goods and services can be produced with ease, as is witnessed in technologically advanced societies. Work, moreover, is essential to our well-being as humans.

A survey of older Americans showed that 40% of men and women between the ages of 50–75 years were working or planned to work in retirement.[2] Another 40% served as volunteers or planned to volunteer when they retired. They did not want a full-time job, but they wanted to work and make a contribution in the larger scheme of society. Apparently, for many, the need to work does not automatically disappear at the age of retirement. They may quit their jobs, but they do not stop working.

KEY POINT

Work serves many purposes, among them providing necessary and useful materials and services, an opportunity for service, and—in cooperation with others—an opportunity to build community and a means to use and develop individual gifts and talents.

Positive Work Experiences

You probably have experienced the joys of work at one time or another, whether in a job for which you receive wages or in doing a household chore, such as cleaning your house or raking the yard. You drew satisfaction not just from the results of the work (a job well done or a clean house or yard) but also from the process. You inherently know what work is good regardless of what others may think.

Perhaps your work is not separated from the rest of life but permeates your entire manner of living. You see work a useful endeavor that is satisfying in itself and brings significant pleasure. Such work is an important part of a harmonious life and is not viewed as a duty or an obsession.

A positive attitude toward work contributes to a harmonious life–work spirit state. Some of the qualities that contribute to a positive work attitude are described in Exhibit 10-1. People who display these qualities consider whatever work they are engaged in to be part of a greater whole. Their sense of purpose is not obscured by a particular task so they can shift their thinking and actions as needed. In the interests of furthering a project, they will put aside what they are doing to help a coworker when necessary.

- They see the unifying patterns and common threads, not just the conflicts and contradictions.
- They perceive the possibilities and draw on varied resources instead of becoming mired in old mindsets.
- They recognize and appreciate the contributions and talents of their coworkers.
- They measure their effectiveness by the quality of their relationships.
- They delight in the work process as well as the product.
- They possess an enthusiasm in the work setting that suggests harmony of spirit and optimum balance of life and work.

EXHIBIT 10-1   Qualities Consistent with a Positive Work Attitude

A person with a positive work attitude

- Is rejuvenated rather than depleted by work
- Gives full attention to the effort
- Experiences an altered sense of time
- Displays a creative and nurturing outlook
- Is optimistic
- Demonstrates open-mindedness
- Has abundant energy
- Feels a sense of purpose
- Sees self as an important contributor to a great order
- Appreciates the contributions of others

Negative Work Experiences

Not everyone in today's society experiences harmony in their life and work. Job stress seems to be a common problem in all industrialized societies. Unemployment, underemployment, and overwork are major problems.

Work is commonly seen in negative terms in our modern industrial society. In the interests of efficiency, jobs sometimes are limited to a small segment of a task that does not afford us a sense of the whole. Our language reflects this idea. People are called "cogs in the wheels of industry" or a "minor functionary in the machinery of an organization," and compared with computers, their effectiveness is measured by their ability to multitask. Work becomes misdirected and no longer serves our purposes. Instead, work creates undue stress and absorbs an undue portion of our attention.

Unemployment

For those who are unemployed, the lack of work can have profound emotional and spiritual effects. These people are deprived of an opportunity to realize their unique talents, to contribute to the welfare of their families, and to pay taxes that will service the greater community. When they are forced to depend on public assistance for extended periods of time, their pride is further undermined. They receive the message that they are not needed or valued and in some measure almost become invisible.

Unemployment certainly affects society in more than an economic sense. The unemployed are unable to fully participate in the community. Is it in any wonder that people who are not able to contribute through working turn to violence, drugs, and other modes of self-hatred as a way of announcing their presence? Everyone needs a sense of feeling needed and making a contribution to the welfare of others within the scope of their capability.

Underemployment

Underemployment, although perhaps not as clearly harmful as unemployment, also takes a toll on the persons affected. The message for the underemployed, although more subtle, is the same as for the unemployed. Some may derive limited satisfaction from being gainfully occupied and perhaps being able to pay bills. They often work in part-time jobs or only part of the year when they want full-time employment year round. They believe they have no options, and thus, they stay in their jobs. Still others remain in jobs that do not truly engage them simply because they earn high wages. They turn to activities other than work for fulfillment or seek pleasure in what their wages can buy them. They may work in jobs that require little skill and afford almost no chance to develop any of their special talents or realize personal achievements.

Overwork

Overwork is an increasing problem. Sometimes this addiction to work is driven by the desire for consumer goods. Nothing is good enough; there is always a better appliance or gadget to lure us, and these new and improved objects cost money. It is easy to get caught in the wheel of earning and spending. As we increase the time devoted to work, we often sacrifice health, relationships, and other important areas of our lives. We spend so much time earning money to buy things that we seldom get to enjoy what we have bought.

KEY POINT

There is a perception that people are killing themselves with work, busyness, and multitasking. Workaholism is a modern epidemic that is sweeping our land.

Some of us become workaholics whereby our fundamental identities are equated with our work; we see ourselves only in terms of our jobs: "I am an accountant," or "I am a lawyer." Success is solely measured by the number of clients or cases and/or the amount of money earned. Workaholics have difficulty relaxing. There is a persistent need to complete a few more tasks before they can feel good and allow themselves a break. At the same time, they often feel resentful about their need to continue their frantic, compulsive working. If anything happens to prevent them from continuing this pattern, their basic identity is threatened. Being is completely absorbed by doing.

Even when performing acts of charity, workaholics press on to do more and more. Guilt drives them on, never allowing them to rest.

KEY POINT

Overwork is toxic, whatever the goal, because it separates us from our deeper selves and unbalances us.

Disconnection

Many people have separated their lives from their work and endure work in order to satisfy materialistic needs and desires. They dream of retirement when they can be free of the burden of work. Work is not a natural part of their lives.

Work for many is experienced in jobs that mostly consist of mindless and repetitive tasks for which they have little interest that are designed to produce profits for which they have little shares. Discontent, passiveness, boredom, lack of joy, a sense of hopelessness, and a vague feeling that life is meaningless permeates these situations.

Values Conflict

Sometimes the values of the organizations people work for conflict with their personal values. For example, a salesperson may believe that honesty is important and takes care to avoid being dishonest in his personal interactions. The company the salesperson represents may have the practice of convincing people they cannot obtain the product through any other source when, in fact, there are other distributors of the product. The salesperson may struggle between being dishonest to customers or telling the truth and not getting the sale—or even losing his job. This type of conflict also can arise when a nurse who is Christian and holds the belief that abortion is morally wrong works in a clinic that counsels and refers pregnant women for abortions. In some circumstances, people can avoid or leave jobs that place them in such conflicts, but sometimes, that option is not possible.

Organizational Changes

Fortunately, there is emerging awareness that job situations that are fragmented and disconnected from a sense of the whole are not only disadvantageous for the workers, but also not good for the bottom line either. Flexible hours, child care, parent leave, and job sharing are helpful in some cases but do not serve most workers. Current trends of increasing burnout, decreased employee satisfaction, and rising healthcare costs are spurring changes in work settings. Greater attention is being paid to how an organization can improve the quality of work for employees, not just how employees can benefit the organization. New models for organizations that emphasize balance are being tried.

KEY POINT

Organizations, like individuals, need to achieve a balance between input and output. Like fossil fuels, individuals and organizations need to be replenished.

What Is to Be Done?

The problems associated with work in today's society are very complex. Thus, what can be done? The achievement of harmony and balance in work and life occurs when life and livelihood are reunited. People need to search for ways to convert negative work experiences into positive ones. This begins with them taking the first step by changing their image of work.

Some people may have given little thought to the full impact and image of work in their lives. They may think of work in terms of a paycheck and benefits and productivity for the employer. In order for them to achieve a healthier work life, they need to reflect on the quality of their work experience. Exhibit 10-2 offers a Spirituality of Work Questionnaire that can be used to guide people through this process. The response can be used as a springboard for discussion leading to a deeper exploration of the meaning of work.

EXHIBIT 10-2   Spirituality of Work Questionnaire

1. Do you feel drawn to the work you do? If yes, why did you choose this work? Has this feeling increased or decreased over time? Why?
2. Do you have a sense of purpose in the work you do?
3. Do you experience your work as a part of a greater whole?
4. What are the unifying patterns in your work?
5. Do you experience enthusiasm for your work? If so, under what circumstances? How frequently? What increases your enthusiasm? What dampens it?
6. How does your work enhance or interfere with your creative expression?
7. Do you continue to learn from your work? Why or why not?
8. How does your work affect others?
9. Who benefits from your work?
10. In what ways does your work distress others?
11. How do you recognize the talents and contributions of others in your work setting?
12. What is the quality of your relationship with coworkers?
13. How does your work affect the environment?
14. Is your work in harmony with the environment?
15. How does your work contribute to caring for the environment?
16. How will your work affect future generations?
17. What are the long-term effects of the work you do?
18. What are the unintended consequences of the work you do?
19. Would you continue to work if you suddenly became independently wealthy? What would you do instead of the work you are now doing? How would you use the money?
20. How do you rest from work and renew yourself?
21. What do you do with your leisure time?
22. What would you do if you had a sabbatical year?
23. What is sacred about the work you do?
24. What is your philosophy of work?
25. What do you value about your work?

What Our Language Tells Us

Our language reflects the time pressure many of us feel on a regular basis. Phrases, such as *time savers, fast food, express lane, rapid transit, overnight delivery,* and *instant message* control our lives. Colleges and universities have created accelerated programs so that students can complete the requirements for a baccalaureate in 3 rather than 4 years and even begin working for a graduate degree while still an undergraduate. Young children are pressured to get a head start in our highly competitive world. Parents rush around shuttling their children to gymnastics, soccer games, computer classes, and other assorted activities to ensure their admission to the better colleges. Free play is almost a thing of the past. We even have an expression for this need to hurry; we say we are experiencing a "time crunch." It is as though things are out of control and we are all traveling at warp speed.

> **REFLECTION**
>
> Notice how your life is affected by the messages that link a fast pace and busyness with importance. What do they do to you? Uncover, accept, and understand the patterns that influence your life. As you increase your awareness of these patterns, you will be in a better position to correct the imbalances you find.

The popular press offers many articles on how to cope with our accelerated pace and be more efficient. We are inundated with suggestions for setting goals, improving organization, and increasing efficiency. We are told, for example, to handle each piece of mail only once, to make lists and prioritize tasks, and to reduce the time in meetings by allotting specific, limited times for each item on the agenda. We are encouraged to speed read and are inundated with periodicals that provide digests of the literature of journals in our fields.

The motto in many work settings is this: "Do more with less and do it faster." Workers sometimes feel that they are treated like parts of a machine, and they must maintain the expected pace or be discarded as obsolete. Although some of the ideas can be helpful, there is the danger of over-planning and structuring life at the expense of living life.

The material and psychological rewards people receive from their increased efficiency may simply prompt them to invest more time and energy into work at the expense of their health, family, and community. They may end up working more efficiently, but also longer hours. Workers in the United States already work more hours than workers in other industrialized countries. It is easier to become psychologically trapped by success as success begets greater expectations for performance.

REFLECTION

Reflect on your own work situation and consider what you can change to promote balance. Reestablish control of your life and schedule. You may need to review your spending habits and eliminate expenses that are not essential in order to reduce the amount of time you spend working. Avoid turning to shopping as therapy. Consider decommercializing holiday festivities and creating simpler but meaningful holiday rituals. Find ways of sharing with your neighbors through borrowing and lending. Practice saying "no." Restore the practice of providing Sabbath time for yourself. You may discover increased life satisfaction!

Balancing Work and Life

People are encouraged to live a balanced life. What, however, is a *balanced life*? *Balance* means the harmonious ratio between all parts, not necessarily equally divided parts. Just as people need to balance the time that they devote to sleep with the time they are awake, they need to balance the time spent in work with the time spent in other activities. Individuals determine this balance for themselves. The ratio of time spent in each activity creates a harmonious whole for them and fosters their well-being.

People need to be challenged with this question: "Why do you work?" All activities—sleeping, eating, playing, and working—are part of living. Work is not something done merely to acquire something else. Work should be connected to one's being and be its expression; it is a *spiritual activity*. Work that is externally driven interferes with that connection.

KEY POINT

Work should serve a higher purpose than merely as the means to acquiring material goods.

Converting Negative into Positive Work Experiences

There is much talk about stress and its effects on health. Some believe stress causes illness and should be decreased, if not totally eliminated. This is an oversimplification of the notion of stress. Stress is inevitable and can be a positive force. Stress, for example, can prompt you to look for solutions and solve problems.

Any number of events that people experience as normal—changes in living conditions, work, relationships, even ordinarily joyous occasions such as marriage or the birth of a child—can be stressful. These stressors, however, do not inevitably cause illness. People can learn to manage them by finding balance with nutrition, exercise, play, and relaxation.

KEY POINT

Humans have varied natural, biologic rhythms like those found in nature. One of the important rhythms humans experience during one 24-hour period is known as the *ultradian rhythm*.
The general pattern of this rhythm is 90 to 120 minutes of activity, followed by a 20-minute
recovery period. Periods of higher energy regularly alternate with signals suggesting a need for
rest. Ignoring signals calling for rest while continuing to work will upset the ultradian rhythm
and lead to stress. Responding appropriately to the call for rest supports the normal pattern
and allows for recovery and renewal. Even a small change in activity may be beneficial. Planning your work so that after approximately 90 minutes of concentration on a project you take
a stretch break or engage in a different activity will help. A play break during work may help to
restore us.

Life-Balancing Skills

Although major problems associated with work can only be addressed on a societal level,
some things can be done to manage many of the problems on an individual basis. Individuals have inner resources that can be drawn upon to cope with daily stresses. Researchers
have found that certain personality traits help people cope effectively with emotional wear
and tear. These traits prevent people from breaking down emotionally and physically in
the face of life crises.

The capacity to *attend*, *connect*, and *express* (ACE factor) feelings can help people to maintain physical and mental health. Feelings (emotions) are gifts that provide people with
information about the effects of what is happening at that moment. When people attend
to those feelings, connect them to consciousness, and express them appropriately, they are
able to cope successfully with stress and restore balance to their systems. For instance, when
you notice a dull, aching pain in your right shoulder, you draw your attention to the pain
(attend) rather than simply try to mask the pain with medication. You ask yourself questions to connect the pain with what is happening to you. When did the pain start? Can the
pain be associated with a particular activity or movement? Is the pain worse at the end of
the work day or work month? What about when the weather is cold or damp? What is the
character of the pain? Does it come on suddenly or does it build up gradually over time? You
may immediately recognize that the pain is related to the increased time you spend at the
computer doing billing before the end of the month. A closer look at how you arrange your
work area may suggest that you are stressing your right shoulder. You notice that you are
repeatedly twisting your right shoulder as you do this monthly task. You are now in the
position to look for creative solutions to your problem. You may realize that you can
rearrange your work station to avoid the stress on your right shoulder. By doing so, you
eliminate the source of your pain and still fulfill your job responsibilities.

Other troubles in the workplace can occur. Work can be a place of misunderstanding or undue competition that threatens well-being. Perhaps your work situation causes irritation or even anxiety. Skill in using the ACE factor can be helpful in such situations. For example, you notice that you tend to make mistakes when you are assigned to work with a particular coworker. The same thing does not happen when you work with others. You feel that this one person does not like you; he or she acts unfriendly and seems to be impatient when things do not go smoothly. You notice that as soon as you receive your assignment to this coworker, your stomach seems to get tied up in knots, and you already sense that things will not go well. You may get stuck in blaming this coworker for your difficulties, complain to your supervisor or union, and/or do all in your power to discredit this person. You may be successful in changing the situation; you or the targeted coworker may be reassigned. You may find you are forced to work with someone who is even more difficult and the situation may grow worse. Now you are faced with an even bigger problem. You are reluctant to call attention to the problem for fear of being labeled "difficult." Your anxiety increases, and you find that your health deteriorates as a result. The ACE factor can be applied in this circumstance as well. You start to attend to the signs that your anxiety level is increasing. You connect the increased anxiety to your tendency to make errors. You acknowledge (express) the link between your anxiety and errors. Your awareness allows you to take steps to reduce your anxiety (e.g., take a few deep breaths). You may further consider the link and discover the underlying source of the anxiety. This coworker works at a faster speed than you do, and your anxiety increases when you cannot match his speed. You ask your coworker for help and you work together to find a solution to the problem.

KEY POINT

The ACE factor can be good for your health. Research shows that people who lack the ACE factor have weaker immune systems, which results in less ability to defend against infectious diseases and cancer. Persons who have greater ACE abilities have stronger immune systems. Quite simply, neither the presence or absence of anxiety nor the degrees of anxiety are the deciding factors. Rather, it is how the person deals with the anxiety that makes the difference.[3,4]

You cannot ignore feelings, disregard their meanings, and repress expression without adverse consequences to your health. Anxiety, like pain, is a signal that tells us something is wrong and needs our attention.

People who are psychologically hardy have been found to have certain characteristics referred to as the three Cs: *commitment, control,* and *challenge.*[5] People who are strong in commitment find meaning and purpose in their work as long as the work is useful and not harmful. They are wholeheartedly involved in whatever work they do. A person who works as a garbage collector, by knowing the meaning of his or her work and appreciating its contribution to society, has commitment. Drudgery may be part of the work, but drudgery does not negate its purpose or value. When we are committed, the meaning of our work will be present to us even when it is obscured by routine and only breaks through to our awareness from time to time.

REFLECTION

Do you feel you have control over your work activities, are committed to them, and are able to framework problems as challenges to overcome rather than threats?

People who believe and behave as though they have influence over life circumstances demonstrate control. These people have a sense of mastery and confidence in their ability to deal with the challenges of life even when faced with limitations in external freedom. Their sense of control is healthy and should be distinguished from unhealthy attempts to control others' behavior and reactions. People who demonstrate control respond to reports that there will be major layoffs in their plant with plans for dealing with that possibility. They begin to make immediate changes in their lifestyles to set aside extra money in the event that they are among those laid off. They do not spend their energy railing against events over which they have no control.

People who are high in challenge view problems resulting from change as trials to overcome and not as threats. These people recognize that change also represents opportunities for growth and not just loss of comfort and security. They creatively adapt to the fact that they may lose their job by exploring other employment possibilities. These are the people who usually have an exit plan in place before they receive their pink slip.

Commitment, control, and challenge, often referred to as the hardiness factors, are the building blocks of healthy coping. Healthy copers respond to loss, instability, and change by drawing on their own inner resources. Those who have the hardiness factor are not necessarily younger, wealthier, better educated, or in possession of greater social support.

People ought not to postpone living because of their work or because of their plans to buy something with the money they make. It is easy to become absorbed in acquiring more and more money and lose sight of the original goal. Exhibit 10-3 lists questions that people can use to gain insight into their work/life balance. It can prove useful for people to discuss their responses with significant others in their lives or a professional who can assist them in making changes.

Downshifting is one response to these daily realities. People find that by working less they are able to do something more meaningful with their lives, including spending more time

---

EXHIBIT 10-3   Questions to Use in Guiding Assessment of Life/Work Balance

· Are you doing that which energizes and renews you?

· What gives you the greatest joy?

· Do you continue to expand your business in response to the opportunity to make more money to the detriment of your health and personal life?

· Do you devote more time to work in order to escape problems at home?

· Do you spend wastefully and then work overtime to pay your bills?

· How would you really like to spend your time?

· What are the things you always wanted to do but do not because of lack of time? How can you find the time to do these things?

---

with their children. This requires a change in their basic thinking. A common tendency is to acquire things that allow us to live more luxuriously but that do not necessarily enhance our lives. These possessions can become anchors that hold us down rather than free us. A person may buy a boat with the dream of spending sunny days relaxing on the water; however, the reality of the attention a boat needs may soon hit. The person will either have to invest time and energy to maintain the boat or spend money for someone else to do so; either option could impose a burden sufficient to dilute the joy of boat ownership. People need to ask themselves whether their purchases will enhance the quality of their lives or be added burdens. Perhaps trips to the local public beach with family and friends could provide equal or greater pleasure than owning a boat.

It is difficult, however, for people to resist the predominant culture on their own. Adjusting to a reduced income requires adjusting to decreased spending. One need not drop out of society to achieve the goal of simplicity. Refusing to buy name brand clothes for their children can initially create conflict for parents. Deciding to reduce spending on holiday presents and celebrations takes courage. Joining a group with similar goals can provide much needed support in efforts to downshift. Newsletters, Web sites, and study circles are springing up around the country to help those interested in transforming their work lives, spending habits, and values to create life/work balance. A list of suggested Web sites is provided at the end of this chapter.

Work is part of your life, but people should not live to work. They need to be careful not to postpone living in order to work. Work life needs to be in balance with personal life in a way that causes people to experience a unity that celebrates their personhood. Current lifestyle habits need not be permanent. People need to ask the critical questions that will help them to create a harmonious life–work balance in their lives.

Summary

Work serves many purposes, including providing materials and services, offering services to others for the purpose of building community, and enabling people to use and develop their gifts and talents. A positive work attitude contributes to a harmonious life–work spirit state and is reflected by being rejuvenated rather than depleted by work, giving full attention to the effort, experiencing an altered sense of time, displaying a creative and nurturing outlook, showing optimism, having abundant energy, demonstrating open-mindedness, feeling a sense of purpose, seeing self as an important contributor to a greater order, and appreciating the contributions of others.

Negative work experiences include unemployment, underemployment, and overwork. Some ways to convert negative work experiences into positive ones include rearranging work schedules to coincide with ultradian rhythm, being attentive to feelings, developing psychological hardiness, and downshifting. People can achieve a higher quality of life by making work a meaningful, but not all-consuming experience.

References

1. Fox, M. (1995). *The Reinvention of Work*. San Francisco: Harper, p. 1.
2. Geary, L. H. (2007). Work until you die: A new retirement goal. *Financial literacy 2007*. Accessed August 6, 2008 from www.bankrate.com/brm/news/Financial_Literacy/April07_retirement_poll_national_a1.asp
3. MacEoin, B. (2008). *Boost Your Immune System Naturally: A Lifestyle Action Plan for Strengthening Your Natural Defenses*. London: Carlton Books.
4. Dreher, H. (1995). *The Immune Power Personality*. New York: Penguin Books, p. 51.
5. Dreher, H. (1995). *The Immune Power Personality*. New York: Penguin Books, p. 52.

Suggested Reading

Aron, C. S. (2001). *Working at Play*. New York: Oxford University Press.

Bolles, R. N. (2007). *What Color Is Your Parachute*. New York: Barnes & Noble.

Briggs, J., & Peat, D. (2000). *Seven Life Lessons of Chaos*. New York: Harper-Perennial.

Caproni, P. J. (2000). *The Practical Coach: Management Skills for Everyday Life*. New York: Pearson Education.

Damasio, A. (2000). *The Feeling of What Happens*. New York: Harcourt, Brace.

Davidson, J., & Dreher, H. (2004). *The Anxiety Book*. New York: Penguin Putnam.

Dossey, B. M., Keegan, L., & Guzzetta, C. E. (2005). *Holistic Nursing* (4th ed.). Sudbury, MA: Jones and Bartlett.

Fassel, D. (2000). *Working Ourselves to Death. The High Cost of Workaholism. The Rewards of Recovery*. San Francisco: iUniverse.

Robinson, J. (2003). *Work to Live: The Guide to Getting a Life*. New York: Perigee.

Rutledge, T. (2002). *Embracing Fear*. New York: HarperCollins.

Swenson, R., & Margin, A. (2002). *The Overload Syndrome*. Colorado Springs: NAV Press.

Wheatley, M. J. (2006). *Leadership and the New Science*. San Francisco: Berrett-Koehler.

Chapter 11

Creative Financial Health

OBJECTIVES

This chapter should enable you to

- · Define money
- · Discuss the energetic principles of money
- · Describe the universal laws that apply to money
- · Discuss the difference between a mechanistic and holistic perspective on money
- · List at least six measures that can promote harmony of body, mind, and spirit in achieving financial goals

Except for the payment of services, the area of finances is rarely regarded as a matter of concern in health care, yet it can significantly influence health status. Money affects all areas of life, including where you live, your education, the types of food you eat, and the amount of stress in your life.

It seems that everywhere you turn you are faced with television programs, articles, and seminars that correlate money with health and happiness. In actuality, there is truth to this. The emerging medical specialty of *psychoneuroimmunology* is confirming that positive emotions and happiness result in a higher functioning immune system and, consequently, better health. If the amount of money you have is responsible for your level of happiness and contentment in life, then you could surmise that money is an important factor in promoting health.

KEY POINT

Minted coins first appeared about 650 B.C. in Asia Minor. The neighboring Greeks began minting coins soon thereafter and within a few centuries developed a system of banking that included borrowing and lending money.

What Is Money?

Money is defined as standard pieces of gold, silver, copper, and nickel used as a medium of exchange. The word money is derived from the Latin word *moneta*, which means mint. One of the definitions of mint is to create, and thus, you could reason that money serves to create. Money often is referred to as *currency*, in which it shares a definition with electricity.

You may think of money in terms of paper and coins that carry value, but it is more than that. Money is an energy that is neutral. Your consciousness gives money the charge, either negative or positive, resulting in how it serves your life. Just as your mind can affect your physical health, it also can affect your financial health.

KEY POINT

There is a common view among spiritual and conscious prosperity coaches that suggests that if all of the wealth in the world were distributed evenly to every man and woman, within a short time period, the rich would be rich and the poor would be poor again.

Beliefs About Money

What is wealth? Who is rich? How do you determine financial security? The answers are based on perceptions, and your belief system creates your perceptual field. Beliefs are derived from a variety of sources, such as societal and cultural influences, religious background, ancestral heritage, educational systems, and the mindset of the adult household in which you were raised. Beliefs about money influence how you manage and use it and how much you have. For example, many people who carry negative beliefs about money find themselves in states of financial deficit and struggle.

Many cultural influences shape beliefs about money. For example, your work ethic conveys the message that "you have to work very hard and struggle for all your money." Certain religious views imply that "to be spiritual one must live in poverty." These views are very old and embedded into masses of minds and consciousness. What messages have influenced your views about money? An awakening moment can come when you gain an understanding of the factors that have contributed to the beliefs you hold about money.

REFLECTION

What does financial security mean to you? How did you develop your beliefs about this?

It may be difficult to identify your true beliefs about money. A good way to discover your beliefs is to observe your thoughts, feelings, emotions, and desires when in the act of a financial exchange. For example, when writing a check to pay a bill or giving a donation, what are your thoughts and feelings? People who see the glass as half empty often find themselves with ongoing thoughts, such as "I can't really afford this," or "I wish I had more." Emotions that often accompany these thoughts can be anger, fear, or guilt; they come from a negative perspective. The good news is that it is possible to change beliefs to heal the wounds of *scarcity consciousness* and move into a more positive place by acquiring *abundance consciousness.*

Energetic Principles of Money

As mentioned, money often is identified as currency, representing an avenue in which electricity or energy flows. Currency also carries a charge (another electrical/energetic term that has been adapted in our monetary transactions) that is given to it by the substance through which it is flowing. The way this applies to the way you deal with money is that the charge comes from your beliefs and attitudes (negative or positive). This charge magnetizes your energy field (through which you view the world), and consequently, through the use of universal law (definition and description to follow), you can put an energetic charge on money with your intentions and thoughts.

Become aware of the thoughts and intentions you have while you are handling money. If you note that they are negative, plan to create a change in your mindset. One suggestion is to have a positive thought or consider your blessings each time that money passes through your hands. Gratitude is always a good energy to instill into money.

Energy masters from the East (who work with energy for healing) teach their students how to handle the physical aspects of money (bills, coins, checks, etc.). They instruct the handling of money to be done with energetic regard to help it flow more easily in one's life. For example, they advise that money should not be folded or stuffed in one's pocket or wallet, but instead placed properly in order with the bills facing in the same direction.

Money as Spiritual Energy

KEY POINT

Money's spiritual roots are represented in its physical form of the dollar bill. On the dollar bill is an eagle that holds in its beak a scroll that reads *E pluribus unum*, which in Latin means *From many, one*. Also pictured on the bill is a pyramid, which is a noted spiritual geometric structure that has a truncated tip that holds the all-seeing eye of the Divine Providence, the guiding power of the universe, and the motto *Annuit coeptis*, which means *He has smiled on our undertakings*. Below the pyramid is a scroll that bears the inscription *Novus ordo seclorum*, which is translated as *new order of the ages*. On every bill we read *In God We Trust*.

Many people who are seeking ways to develop an abundance consciousness use the affirmations, prayers, and other wisdom offered in ancient religious texts. For example, an ancient Hebrew prosperity affirmation is *Jehovah-Jireh, the Lord now richly provides*. In Deuteronomy 8:18, the insight that God is the source of prosperity is conveyed in these words: "You shall remember the Lord your God, for it is he who gives you your power to get wealth." The biblical admonition that "the love of money is the root of all evil" does not imply that money in itself is bad and harmful, but that the love or worship of money is. It is how people use money that matters. A healthy spiritual perspective realizes that money has its place and that it should not be idolized or used to harm others.

REFLECTION

Money can represent many things in a person's life. What does it mean to you?

Money as Metaphor

As money is a formless substance, it can take on various meanings in your life and represent different things. To many people, the degree to which one is loved and cared for is demonstrated with money. Money can represent something that has authority over you or that can be used as a means to control others. Also, the way in which you deal with your money is a reflection of how you take care of yourself. Money is an extension of who you are in all areas of your life; therefore, it is important when taking a holistic view of self and others that money be an integral consideration. The more ways in which this aspect is integrated and seen as a metaphor for different parts of yourself, the more you can come into your wholeness.

Universal Laws

KEY POINT

Universal laws are unbreakable, unchangeable principles that operate in all phases of our lives and existence, for all people everywhere all the time; they are impartial, irrefutable, and unavoidable.

Universal laws are the framework in which you can operate as you change the perspective of money in your life, especially if there is an interest in working on the co-creative process of manifesting more money in your life. In actuality, universal laws exist whether you know about them or not—or whether you choose to work with them or not. They are similar to many physical laws that operate in your daily life of which you may not be aware—such as the law of gravity. Universal laws are nonphysical in nature, but they are fundamental laws of mind and spirit. Everyday life is based on these laws, much like physical laws and laws of nature (changing of seasons, the sun shining, turning on a light switch, taking a shower, and listening to the radio). As you rely on these laws in the physical world, so can you rely on universal laws of mind and spirit. People who consciously work in harmony with these laws find a high degree of fulfillment because they begin to align their actions with their purpose in life.

KEY POINT

Florence Nightingale wrote extensively about universal law in an attempt to unify science and religion in a way that would bring order, meaning, and purpose to human life. She was motivated to use this information to help the working class people of England who wanted and needed an alternative to atheism. Nightingale said that universal laws are expressions of God's thoughts and that law is a continuous manifestation of God's presence.

How Universal Laws Work

Universal laws work on an energetic premise with simple, subtle energy principles. There are two energetic fields in operation, coexisting and intermingling: the universal energy field and the human energy field. The divine order of energy is often referred to as God and is fixed. The human energy field, resulting from beliefs, thoughts, and attitudes, is a mutable force that can be created and formed (the free-will aspect). That which you carry in your human energy field in the form of beliefs, attitudes, and thoughts will create an energetic charge that will incur a response according to universal laws. You can charge your field with new beliefs, attitudes, and thoughts simply by bringing in new input in the form of thoughts, much like one would program information into a computer. The following examples of universal laws will help to further explain how they work.

The Law of Expectancy

The Law of Expectancy suggests that whatever you expect you will receive. This is not the same as wishful thinking, but rather something that is expected with certainty, much like a pregnant woman is expecting a baby. The degree of expectancy that is maintained in your consciousness is vital. What is it that you are expecting? Do you expect to go to work tomorrow? Do you expect to make a certain amount of money? Expectations can limit you, even when you learn to temper your expectations. It is suggested that when working with the Law of Expectancy an open-ended thought should always be maintained; for example, "this or something better" or "this or something more."

Faith is an important element in the Law of Expectancy. This wisdom is reflected in Matthew 9:29 where it is said "according to your faith be it done unto you." In working with this law, it is important not to limit expectations. Imagination helps with that. That is why Einstein said that imagination is more powerful than knowledge.

KEY POINT

Working with the Law of Expectancy is similar to working with principles of the reemerging ancient art of Chinese placement called Feng Shui. Feng Shui is an energetic approach to improving all aspects of one's life by working with the physical space in which people spend most of their time—either at home or in their offices. In Feng Shui, a BaGua is a map used of physical space. The BaGua is a standard template that has in it all areas of one's life and the location in their physical space that is connected to these areas of life. The section of the BaGua that is connected to money is in the Fortunate Blessings location. If there is junk, clutter, or physical discord in this area of someone's home or office, then that may impede the flow of financial energy in one's life. A way to enhance financial abundance in one's life is to clear the physical space in this area of their home according to the BaGua so as to prepare for the flow of blessings and prosperity.

The Law of Preparation

When you prepare for something, you often get it, and that includes negative things as well positive ones. Do you know people who have put money away for a rainy day or an emergency? In a sense, they are preparing for these negative experiences. The energy can be shifted, and instead, they could consider preparing for abundance and success. It is important to prepare for something in your consciousness and then take action to achieve it.

The Law of Forgiveness

Energetically, forgiveness helps to remove blocks to receiving. It releases negative experiences in your consciousness and creates space that allows the entrance of divine consciousness in the form of abundance. One of the country's leading prosperity coaches, Edwene Gaines,[1] believes that all financial debt is about unforgiveness of past issues and, mostly, not forgiving ourselves. She teaches that one of the fastest ways to prosperity and abundance is forgiving on a daily basis. Everyone and everything in the past should be forgiven so as to move forward in one's life abundantly.

REFLECTION

Who and what do you need to forgive?

The Law of Tithing

The word *tithe* means one-tenth and usually is related to offering a portion of income to spiritual or sacred purposes. A tithe is usually given to a person, place, or institution that contributes to one's spiritual nourishment and growth. Tithing is one of the fundamental laws of life and is a powerful prospering exercise. It is an ancient, spiritual practice mentioned throughout the Bible. In Genesis 28:20, Jacob said of "all that Thou shalt give me, I will surely give one-tenth unto Thee." Tithing can be seen as simple as the inflow/outflow principle. As with breathing, where it is necessary to regularly rid yourself of air in order to receive fresh air into the lungs, so it is necessary to give regularly if you wish to receive regularly. "Whatsoever a man soweth, that shall he also reap." If you do not sow, you do not reap.

KEY POINT

The intent with tithing is to plant a seed. A farmer tithes in order to reap harvest, returning one-tenth of the grain to the soil.

Your Mission Becomes Your Money

Every person on this planet has a mission and a purpose in this lifetime. In order to fulfill your destiny, this work (work in the sense of contribution to the world not the source of a paycheck, although it may be delivered in that form) needs to be carried out. Too often, people are not connected to their purpose in life, and consequently, many imbalances may appear, including physical ailments, relationship disputes, and financial difficulties. Financial fulfillment can be derived through the process of following your own heart to perform the work of your dreams. More importantly, by tapping into and executing the right livelihood, spiritual aspects of life can be fulfilled.

The process of discovering your life mission can be a very challenging one. Often, people find themselves going through the motions of a job that not only is ill-suited for them, but may go against many of their natural energetic rhythms; however, the fear of not having enough and not being able to survive compel many to go against their natural flow and tolerate ill-suited work.

REFLECTION

In what ways is your attitude about work different and similar to that of your parents and grandparents?

Discovering your mission in life is a spiritual and creative process. The approach to this process is very simple and begins by exploring your desires. It is that which is your greatest longing that takes you to your mission. Some people spend years not knowing what their purpose in life is, whereas others seem to know their purpose the moment they arrive on the planet. Many job opportunities in our society are focused on the needs of the employer, rather than being designed to fill people's needs of expressing their creative essence and offering their God-given gifts to the world. The system is created in such a way that people end up redesigning themselves to fit the system's needs. This, combined with fears about survival, results in stifled missions. Fear drives people to be stuck in containers (i.e., jobs) that are not made for them.

KEY POINT

A mid-life crisis can occur when people feel they are limited by their jobs and not fulfilling their missions. In this awakening, there is a yearning to follow one's longing. The crisis can result in some unfortunate consequences, such as divorce and unsound business ventures, or in new opportunities that realign with values and life purpose.

Passion Creates Magnetism

There is a vital force connected with fulfilling life purpose and mission. Think of the vitality that people have when they are excited about what they are doing, even if it is interpreted as a mundane act to others. When one is excited, passionate, and satisfied with fulfilling an act of life, there is a certain charge that is being created in the vital force field (energy; electromagnetic field) of the individual. This energy creates magnetism, and this magnetism draws in universal energy, which manifests abundance.

Fulfilling Mission versus Collecting a Paycheck

Identifying your mission is integral to the process of attaining financial balance that leads to wealth and abundance, but equally important are the implementation and action. There is a popular confusion with work being defined as paid employment. By expanding your thinking to defining work as any activity from which you derive purpose, fulfillment, and meaning—rather than limiting the view of work to paid employment—you can begin to value your activities and yourself differently.

Being limited in your ability to express your mission because of needing to meet the employer's agenda potentially can be disempowering to you. It is important to recognize this and allow your own mission to be expressed—even if it is through a hobby or volunteer activity rather than formal employment.

REFLECTION

It is possible that one's mission may not be expressed regularly in the daily place of employment. What are your avenues to expressing your purpose and mission?

From a Mechanistic to a Holistic Perspective on Money

Dealing with money from a physical perspective keeps it in the mechanistic model, which implies that money is a separate entity in and of itself. The making and utilization of money are confined to the physical realm. This suggests that there are no other influences on money other than cause and effect from the physical perspective—work, investments, savings, and budgeting increase available money.

There is another way to view money, however, involving a more holistic view. A crucial principle involved in the holistic paradigm is that nonphysical substance (thought, intention, requests) results in physical matter (physical manifestation of the request). In other words, belief that a goal can be fulfilled can bring about desired results. Spiritual masters have promoted similar beliefs, including Jesus who said, "All things whatsoever ye shall ask in prayer, believing, ye shall receive" (Matthew 21:22).

KEY POINT

The scientific arena of quantum physics aids in understanding how the mind's creative force can manifest itself in the physical world by explaining that rapidly spinning atomic particles are invisible, but slower ones exist in the form of physical matter. Faster spinning particles can slow down and create physical forms. Consistent with this theory, thoughts can be manifested as physical matter.

The nonphysical substance used in this holistic paradigm is a creative force that allows individuals to produce in the physical world that which they are thinking. The creative force within people is not connected to personality or ego; however, it is important to identify the belief systems and perceptions under which personality operates to be aware of barriers that could impede the creative force.

After aligning with purpose, the next step is to focus on the request, desire, or goal that one wants to manifest. It is important to remember to leave results open-ended by adding the words *or something better* to requests. At this point, it can be helpful to visualize what the end result may look like. For example, if you desire a specific amount of money, visualize a bank statement that shows that particular amount as your savings account balance or the exact item you wish to purchase with that amount of money.

EXHIBIT 11-1   Mind, Body, and Spirit Harmony in Achieving Financial Goals

· Recognize that there is a power greater than yourself that can affect your outcomes.

· Quiet your mind, and connect to the creative force of the universe.

· Clarify and align with your purpose and mission in life.

· Consider the ways in which you can share and use your money to benefit other people and purposes.

· State and visualize your desire and specific goal.

· Be aware of emotions connected to financial goals and actions.

· Release preconceived notions of the ways in which resources will be delivered and the forms in which they will come.

· Trust and have faith that your results will be achieved.

· Express gratitude for what you receive.

As it is important to visualize and see in the mind's eye what is desired (see Exhibit 11-1), at the same time, it is important to let go of the process and outcome. Releasing is the last and possibly the most difficult step in the creative manifestation process. The act of releasing the entire process and letting go of the outcome calls one to progress in faith and trust that a greater power will be in control.

We live in a time in which the ways we perceive the world and our lives are changing. We can access information from higher places and pay more attention to the higher senses of our being, such as intuition and belief in the nonphysical world. With this heightening in perspective comes more options and approaches for accessing creative solutions. Money is a representative energy through which we can demonstrate the ability to affect forces in our life and create something out of nothing.

Summary

From a mechanistic view, money is viewed in terms of its physical characteristics; however, from a holistic view, money is more than a medium of exchange to purchase goods and services; it represents an avenue through which energy flows. People's attitudes and beliefs about money and their financial well-being can influence the amount of money they receive and its use. To obtain financial goals successfully, people must have harmony of body, mind, and spirit.

Reference

1. Gaines, E. (2003). *Riches and Honor.* Audiocassette. Valley Head, AL: Prosperity Products. Available from www.prosperityproducts.com.

Suggested Reading

Barnett, E. W., Gordon, L. S., & Hendrix, M. A. (2001). *The Big Book of Presbyterian Stewardship.* Louisville, KY: Geneva Press.

Blomberg, C. (2001). *Neither Poverty or Riches: A Biblical Theology of Possessions.* Grand Rapids, MI: Eerdmans.

Chopra, D. (1998). *Creating Affluence: The A to Z Steps to a Richer Life.* Novato, CA: New World Library.

Chopra, D. (2007). *The Seven Spiritual Laws of Success. A Pocketbook Guide to Fulfilling Your Dreams.* San Rafael, CA: Amber-Allen Publishing.

Dunham, L. (2002). *Graceful Living: Your Faith, Values, and Money in Changing Times.* New York: Reformed Church in America Press.

Gawain, S. (2000). *Creating True Prosperity.* Novato, CA: New World Library.

Haughey, J. C. (1997). *Virtue and Affluence: The Challenge of Wealth.* Kansas City: Sheed & Ward.

Horton, C. (2002). *Consciously Creating Wealth.* Golden, CO: Higher Self Workshops.

Murphy, L., & Nagel, T. (2002). *The Myth of Ownership: Taxes and Justice.* New York: Oxford University Press.

Ponder, C. (2003). *A Prosperity Love Story: Rags to Enrichment.* Camarillo, CA: DeVorss & Co.

Walters, D. J. (2000). *Money Magnetism: How to Attract What You Need When You Need It.* California: Crystal Clarity Publishers.

Chapter 12

Environmental Effects on Health

OBJECTIVES

This chapter should enable you to

- · List at least six symptoms of toxicity
- · List six sources of toxic substances
- · Describe at least four ways that people can reduce environmental risks to the immune system
- · Outline guidelines for detoxification

Everything in the environment—the food that you eat, the air you breathe, the sensations you experience—affects your body, positively or negatively. Maximizing the benefits of the environment, while reducing the negative impact, is important to promoting good health.

Internal and External Environments

You are affected by two types of environments: external and internal. External environment implies anything that is outside your body, such as the weather, elements in the air, food, sounds, and interactions with other people. Major environmental crises such as catastrophic floods, fires, and hurricanes affect you, as do the minor daily crises, such as waiting in long lines at the supermarket or getting stuck in traffic.

Internal environment pertains to that which is inside you. All that you encounter in your daily living is experienced within you and influences your thinking, feelings, and behavior. Often these events produce some degree of stress that you deal with uniquely based on your sensitivity, perception, awareness, flexibility, and adaptability. You use many skills and resources to balance the stressors from your external and internal environments and stay healthy.

REFLECTION

Think about times in your life when your stress levels have been unusually high. Did you find that you had a higher incidence of illness or injury during or after those times?

Immune System

The immune system's primary purpose is to offer protection from infections or illnesses and to fight disease-producing microorganisms, such as bacteria, viruses, and fungi. In other words, the immune system helps to maximize your health potential as well as to maintain your health. The weakening of the immune system frequently results in an increased susceptibility to unpleasant symptoms, illnesses, and diseases. If the immune system is severely weakened or suppressed, it cannot destroy or reprogram the cells in the body. Environmental conditions influence the normal function of the immune system and can threaten its optimum function (see Chapter 5 for a discussion of the immune system).

Toxicity

> **KEY POINT**
>
> The word *toxicity* generally refers to a poisonous, disease-producing substance that is produced by a microorganism.

Toxicity can result from environmental agents that produce poisonous substances that cause an unhealthy environment within the body, leading to physiological or psychological problems. The accumulation of toxins weakens the immune system. Initially, mild symptoms affecting the body organs, such as a headache, sneezing, swollen eyelids, or irritability may be experienced. Other physical symptoms often include fatigue, restlessness, insomnia, difficulty breathing, and confusion. At first, these symptoms are faint and may be missed or minimized; however, when such symptoms continue over an extended period of time, they are difficult to ignore. Toxicity that continues for a long time begins to impede the normal functions of the body's organs and systems. This results in an imbalance, leading to impairments in normal digestion, walking, and thinking.

Heavy Metals

In your daily environment, you are constantly exposed to environmental factors that lead to the development of toxicity in your body. Of these, the major category of toxic substances is heavy metals.

> **KEY POINT**
>
> Toxic substances can be found in a variety of sources, such as heavy metals, chemicals, parasites, pesticides, and radiation.

Aluminum, arsenic, cadmium, lead, and mercury are examples of heavy metals. They are found in air, food, and water and have no function in the human body. Over a long period of time, these heavy metals accumulate in the body and reach toxic levels. Heavy metals tend to accumulate in the brain, kidneys, and immune system, where they can severely disrupt normal functioning. Heavy-metal toxicity causes unusual symptoms and ailments that tend to linger for an extraordinary length of time. People with symptoms related to this toxicity may visit several medical doctors to find out what is wrong, but often physicians are unable to identify and treat the problem. Frequently medications are prescribed for symptomatic relief but may provide minimal to no relief.

Transportation companies, waste management companies, and manufacturers have been major sources of heavy-metal pollution. For example, many manufacturing plants throughout the United States have polluted the air with poisonous toxins, particularly lead, from their industrial processes and productivity. Exhibit 12-1 lists the common sources of the five heavy metals—aluminum, arsenic, cadmium, lead, and mercury.

EXHIBIT 12-1   Common Sources of Heavy Metal Toxins

Type of Toxins	Source	Type of Toxins	Source
Aluminum	Aluminum cookware		Tap water
	Aluminum foil		Toothpaste
	Antacids		
	Antiperspirants	**Arsenic**	Air pollution
	Baking powder (Aluminum containing)		Antibiotics (given to commercial livestock)
	Bleached flour		Bone meal
	Buffered aspirin		Certain marine plants
	Canned acidic foods		Chemical processing
	Cooking utensils		Coal-fired power plants
	Cookware		Defoliants
	Dental amalgams		Dolomite
	Foil		Drinking water
	Food additives		Drying agents for cotton
	Medications—drugs		Fish
	Antidiarrheal agents		Herbicides
	Anti-inflammatory agents		Insecticides
	Hemorrhoid medications		Kelp
	Vaginal douches		Laundry aids
	Processed cheese		Meats (from commercially raised poultry and cattle)
	"Softened" water		Metal ore
	Table salt		

(continues)

EXHIBIT 12-1   Common Sources of Heavy Metal Toxins *(continued)*

Type of Toxins	*Source*	*Type of Toxins*	*Source*
	Pesticides		Sewage sludge
	Seafood (fish, mussels, oysters)		Soft drinks
	Smelting		Soil
	Smog		"Softened" water
	Smoke		Smelting plants
	Specialty glass		Welding fumes
	Table salt	**Lead**	Air pollution
	Tap water		Ammunition (shot and bullets)
	Tobacco		Bathtubs (cast iron, porcelain steel)
	Wood preservatives		
Cadmium	Air pollution		Batteries
	Art supplies		Canned foods
	Bone meal		Ceramics
	Cigarette smoke		Colored advertisements
	Fertilizers		Chemical fertilizers
	Food (coffee, tea, fruits, and vegetables grown in cadmium-laden soil)		Cosmetics
			Dolomite
			Dust
	Freshwater fish		Food grown near industrial areas
	Fungicides		
	Highway dusts		Gasoline
	Incinerators		Hair dyes and rinses
	Meats (kidneys, liver, poultry)		Leaded glass
			Newsprint
	Mining		Paints
	Nickel-cadmium batteries		Pesticides
	Oxide dusts		Pewter
	Paints		Pottery
	Pesticides		Rubber toys
	Phosphate fertilizers		"Softened" water
	Plastics		Solder in tin cans
	Power plants		Tap water
	Refined foods		Tobacco smoke
	Refined grains		
	Seafood (crab, flounder, mussels, oysters, scallops)	**Mercury**	Contaminated fish
			Cosmetics
	Secondhand smoke		Dental fillings

SOURCES: Adapted from Balch & Balch (1997), Marti (1995), Post-Gazette (10/14/99), Pouls (1999), Ronzio (1999).

KEY POINT

Overall the heavy metals tend to[1]

- Decrease the function of the immune system
- Increase allergic reactions
- Alter genetic mutation
- Increase acidity of the blood
- Increase inflammation of arteries and tissues
- Increase hardening of artery walls
- Increase progressive blockage of arteries

Aluminum

The average person ingests between 3 and 10 milligrams of aluminum each day.[2] Of the various sources of aluminum, the highest exposure comes from the chronic consumption of aluminum-containing antacid products. It is primarily absorbed through the digestive tract as well as through the other organs, such as the lungs and skin. Research has suggested that the heavy metal aluminum contributes to neurologic disorders such as Parkinson's disease, dementia, clumsiness of movements, staggering when walking, and the inability to pronounce words properly.[2] Aluminum tends to accumulate in the brain, bones, kidneys, and stomach tissues. Consequently, the common health problems caused by aluminum are colic, irritation of the esophagus, gastroenteritis, kidney damage, liver dysfunction, loss of appetite, loss of balance, muscle pain, dementia, psychosis, seizures, shortness of breath, and general weakness.[2]

Arsenic

Arsenic is another highly toxic substance. It has an affinity for most of the bodily organs, especially the gastrointestinal system, lungs, skin, hair, and nails. In acute arsenic poisoning, nausea and vomiting, bloody urine, muscle cramps, fatigue, hair loss, and convulsions are noted. Headaches, confusion, abdominal pain, burning of the mouth and throat, diarrhea, and drowsiness may occur in chronic arsenic poisoning. Arsenic toxicity can contribute to the development of cancer (lung and skin), coma, neuritis, peripheral vascular (vessels of the extremities) problems, and collapse of blood vessels.[1]

Cadmium

Cadmium is also considered an extremely poisonous heavy metal. Inhaling cadmium fumes causes pulmonary edema, followed by pneumonia and various degrees of lung damage.

Another way that a person can acquire cadmium poisoning is by ingesting foods contaminated by cadmium-plated containers; these cause violent gastrointestinal symptoms. Cadmium levels also arise in individuals who have zinc deficiencies.

KEY POINT

The health problems that can arise from cadmium toxicity are anemia, cancer, depressed immune system response, dry and scaly skin, emphysema, eye damage, fatigue, hair loss, heart disease, hypertension, increased risk of cataract formation, joint pain, kidney stones or damage, liver dysfunction or damage, loss of appetite, loss of sense of smell, pain in the back and legs, and yellow discoloration of the teeth. These problems occur because cadmium tends to gravitate to tissues of specific body organs, including the brain and its pain centers, the heart and its blood vessels, the kidneys, and the lungs, as well as the tissues that influence the appetite.[1]

Lead

Of all of the common heavy metals, lead has attracted public attention since the early 1900s. At the turn of the 20th century, paint companies knew that lead was a serious risk to health; however, they continued to produce building paints that contained a lead base. These paints were used in homes and commercial buildings. Consequently, children were seriously affected by lead poisoning. In addition, the Environmental Protection Agency estimated that drinking water accounts for approximately 20% of young children's lead exposure.[3] Health problems in children caused by lead poisoning include: attention deficit disorder, hyperactivity syndromes, learning disabilities, loss of appetite, low achievement scores, low intelligent quotients, seizures, and, on occasion, death. Because of the public outcry against lead-based paint, it was banned in 1978. At the same time, the government issued regulations cutting out lead in gasoline.

KEY POINT

Research has shown that declines in IQ are associated with higher blood concentrations of lead.[4]

Lead poisoning affects cognitive (intellectual) function. Studies have revealed that low-level lead exposure impairs children's IQ.[4] In addition to the danger for young children, there was also a great risk of harm from lead exposure for infants and pregnant women. In pregnant women, lead toxicity may cause premature birth, miscarriage, and birth defects.

Lead toxicity may produce a variety of additional symptoms, including abdominal pain, anemia, anorexia, anxiety, bone pain, brain damage, coma, confusion, constipation, convulsions, dizziness, drowsiness, fatigue, heart attack, headaches, high blood pressure, inability to concentrate, indigestion, irritability, kidney disease, loss of muscle coordination, memory difficulties, mental depression, mental damage, muscle pain, nervous system, neurological damage, pallor, and vomiting.

Mercury

As Exhibit 12-1 shows, mercury is found in many sources that we use in our daily life. This toxic metal accumulates in the bones, brain, heart, kidneys, liver, nervous system, and pancreas. Some studies have shown a relationship between unusual symptoms and mercury exposure from silver fillings, finding that a major source of mercury toxicity in the human body was the dental filling and when mercury fillings were removed, the symptoms and related health problems disappeared; however, recent research is challenging the claim that mercury fillings are dangerous.[5] Although mercury levels in blood and urine do increase somewhat with amalgam dental fillings, toxic levels apparently do not occur. Elevated urine and hair levels merely reflect the ongoing elimination of mercury from the body by these routes.[5]

Reducing Environmental Risks to Health

Assess

To begin helping yourself, you need to take an objective look at yourself. One method of self-assessment is the Toxicity Self-Test, shown in Exhibit 12-2. It involves checking off symptoms frequently experienced within 15 common areas and the degree to which each symptom has been noticed; then the score is totaled. The final score may fall in the mild, moderate, or severe range, as indicated at the end of the Toxicity Self-Test checklist. After this assessment is completed, you can explore ways of reducing the toxicity that exists in your body. There are daily positive actions that you can take to reduce or prevent the accumulation of toxins in the body.

Attend to the Basics

With the fast pace of life and all the demands of family and work, it is easy to neglect yourself. This negligence affects your sleep, rest, relaxation, and leisure. Reflect on your daily activities and ask: Am I getting adequate rest? Do I awaken feeling refreshed? Am I taking time to relax and enjoy the simple pleasures of life?

It is important to make sure you are getting sufficient water in order to flush toxins from the body. Be sure to drink at least eight glasses of chemical-free water daily.

EXHIBIT 12-2 Toxicity Self-Test

Rate each of the following symptoms based on your health profile for the past 30 days.

Point Scale:

0 = never or almost never have the symptom

1 = occasionally have the symptom; effect is not severe

2 = occasionally have the symptom; effect is severe

3 = frequently have the symptom; effect is not severe

4 = frequently have the symptom; effect is severe

1. Digestive Function
    ___ Nausea or vomiting
    ___ Diarrhea
    ___ Constipation
    ___ Bloated feeling
    ___ Belching, passing gas
    ___ Heartburn
    ___ TOTAL

2. Ears
    ___ Itchy ears
    ___ Earaches, ear infection
    ___ Drainage from ear
    ___ Ringing in ears, hearing loss
    ___ TOTAL

3. Emotions
    ___ Mood swings
    ___ Anxiety, fear, nervousness
    ___ Anger, irritability
    ___ Depression
    ___ TOTAL

4. Energy/Activity
    ___ Fatigue, sluggishness
    ___ Apathy, lethargy
    ___ Hyperactivity

    ___ Restlessness
    ___ TOTAL

5. Eyes
    ___ Watery, itchy eyes
    ___ Swollen, reddened, or sticky eyelids
    ___ Dark circles under eyes
    ___ Blurred vision/tunnel vision
    ___ TOTAL

6. Head
    ___ Headache
    ___ Faintness
    ___ Dizziness
    ___ Insomnia
    ___ TOTAL

7. Lungs
    ___ Chest congestion
    ___ Asthma, bronchitis
    ___ Shortness of breath
    ___ Difficulty breathing
    ___ TOTAL

8. Mind
    ___ Poor memory
    ___ Confusion
    ___ Poor concentration

(continues)

EXHIBIT 12-2 Toxicity Self-Test *(continued)*

___ Poor coordination

___ Difficulty making decisions

___ Stuttering, stammering

___ Slurred speech

___ Learning disabilities

___ TOTAL

9. Mouth/Throat

___ Chronic coughing

___ Gagging, frequent need to clear throat

___ Sore throat, hoarse

___ Swollen or discolored tongue, gums, lips

___ Canker sores

___ TOTAL

10. Nose

___ Stuffy nose

___ Sinus problems

___ Hay fever

___ Sneezing attacks

___ Excessive mucus

___ TOTAL

11. Skin

___ Acne

___ Hives, rash, dry skin

___ Hair loss

___ Flushing or hot flashes

___ Excessive sweating

___ TOTAL

12. Heart

___ Skipped heartbeats

___ Rapid heartbeat

___ Chest pains

___ TOTAL

13. Joints/Muscles

___ Pain or aches in muscles

___ Arthritis

___ Stiffness, limited movement

___ Pain or aches in muscles

___ Feelings of weakness or tiredness

___ TOTAL

14. Weight

___ Binge eating/drinking

___ Craving certain foods

___ Excessive weight

___ Compulsive eating

___ Water retention

___ Underweight

___ TOTAL

15. Other

___ Frequent illness

___ Frequent or urgent urination

___ Genital itch and/or discharge

___ TOTAL

Add the numbers to arrive at a total for each section. Add the totals for each section to arrive at the grand total.

Mild toxicity = 0–96 grand total score

Moderate toxicity = 97–168 grand total score

Severe toxicity = 169–240 grand total score

REFLECTION

Are you drinking at least eight glasses of water daily to flush toxins from your body? How can you assure the water you drink is free from contamination by lead and other chemicals?

Relax

Relaxation can be achieved by using a variety of techniques.

Guided imagery: Investigative findings have revealed a relationship between lowered immune function and health problems. Guided imagery is done by creating mental scenes in one's mind and has been shown helpful in strengthening the immune system. This imagery technique, also known as mental imagery or *visual imagery*, uses the body–mind connection to alleviate energy imbalances in the body.

Meditation: Meditation is the practice and system of thought that incorporates exercises to attain bodily or mental control and well-being, as well as enlightenment. Studies have shown that a relationship exists between meditation and increased immunity. There are several ways to meditate. One person may prefer to meditate to a particular sound, whereas another may focus on breathing. You may need to try a few styles to determine your personal preference.

Deep breathing: Deep breathing, or belly breathing, can promote relaxation. This method is described in Chapter 4.

Get a Massage

Deep-tissue massages or lymph massages are helpful for the release of toxicity and balancing energy. In deep-tissue massage, the therapist applies greater pressure and focuses on deeper muscles than in the Swedish massage, which primarily aims to promote relaxation. The purpose of lymph massage is to increase the circulation throughout the lymphatic system. Through massage of deeper tissues and increased circulation, toxins are mobilized, released, and eventually eliminated from the body. Beware that deep-tissue massage is not recommended for individuals who have high blood pressure, a history of inflammation of the veins, or any other circulatory problem.

Sweat It Out

Engaging in regular saunas can help relieve the body of toxins through the skin. If you choose to use a sauna, it is best to avoid eating within 1 hour before the sauna to avoid nausea.

Brush Your Skin

Another valuable technique is brushing the skin with a dry brush that has firm natural bristles. The purpose of skin brushing is to rid the body of the poisonous substances that are excreted through perspiration.

Use Nutritional Supplements

Specific nutrient supplements can be taken when you are trying to combat heavy metal toxicity:

- Multivitamin supplement
- Vitamin C
- B-complex vitamins
- Mineral supplements, especially calcium, chromium, copper, iron, magnesium, and zinc
- Sulfur-containing amino acids, including cysteine, methionine, and taurine

Detoxify

Another simple method for the general elimination of toxins is cleansing the bowel. This is a form of detoxification therapy.

KEY POINT

Detoxification was strongly recommended by pioneers in nutritional and natural medicine, including Bernard Jensen, John H. Kellogg, Max Gerson, and John Tilden.

Detoxification, a noninvasive process, has been quite popular in many healthcare systems around the world, especially Europe—to a much greater extent than in the United States. Detoxification is essential as a first step in clearing the body of toxicity because a person cannot rebuild nor maintain health if the toxins remain stored in the body. The majority of toxins tend to accumulate in the bowel where waste matter in the intestines remains for lengthy periods of time. This allows the toxins to be absorbed into the bloodstream throughout the body, causing health problems. After the toxins are cleansed out of the bowel, the body can begin to heal itself. Typically, a fiber substance, such as ground flaxseeds or psyllium husks in powdered form is taken to aid the body in eliminating the toxins. Exhibit 12-3 shows the effect of toxins on unhealthy and healthy functions within the body.

EXHIBIT 12-3   Impact of Toxins on Unhealthy and Healthy Functions in the Body

Unhealthy

· Toxins form internally, leak through the unhealthy intestine, and flow to the liver.

· Toxins are not completely detoxified in the unhealthy liver.

· Unchanged toxins leave the liver and are stored in tissues, such as fat, the brain, and the nervous system.

Healthy

· Few toxins are formed, and most of the them are excreted, with only a small amount naturally transported to the liver.

· Toxins are transformed to an intermediate substance.

· The intermediate substance is transformed to a more water soluble substance and released to the kidneys.

· The water soluble substance is excreted via the urine.

Source: Detoxification, San Clemente, CA: Metagenics, Inc. August, 1994.

KEY POINT

General Guidelines for Detoxification

In using the detoxification process, be aware that it must be done slowly. The reason for this is that the body must adapt to the changes that are occurring. If the detoxification occurs rapidly, unusual symptoms can develop because of the bodily changes that are causing an imbalance. If the detoxification is performed at a slower pace, the body develops its equilibrium while it is eliminating the toxins. Following the detoxification, it is generally recommended that you:

· Drink at least 8 ounces of water each day. Water helps the body to get rid of the debris and also provides sufficient liquid to help with elimination.

· Begin eating raw foods, including vegetables. This provides fiber, a natural substance, that helps with rebuilding tissue in the body.

· Continue to avoid eating the foods listed in Exhibit 12-4. The avoidance of the suggested foods will decrease the faulty bowel function that occurs with an imbalanced diet.

EXHIBIT 12-4   Recommended Nutritional Changes to Reduce Toxicity

Avoid the following:

- Alcohol, drugs, cigarettes
- Caffeinated drinks
- Chlorinated (tap) water
- Commercially prepared foods
- Fats
- Foods high in additives and preservatives
- Hydrogenated and partially hydrogenated oils
- Fried foods
- Heated polyunsaturated fats (fast food oils, theater popcorn oil)
- Monosodium glutamate
- Refined sugars
- Soft drinks
- Softened tap water
- Topical oils (cottonseed, palm)
- White flour foods

REFLECTION

What can you do to reduce exposure to toxins?

Contact with environmental pollutants is a reality of daily life. You come in contact with them in the air you breathe, the foods you eat, and the water you drink. These toxic substances can threaten your health in several ways and lead to major health problems such as lung damage, mood changes, neurological dysfunction, tissue damage, and visual disturbances. By avoiding exposure as much as possible and minimizing or eliminating the build-up of toxins within your tissues and organs, you can protect your health and enjoy maximum function. Exhibit 12-5 gives specific suggestions to help avoid exposure to toxicity in our work, homes, and community environments.

EXHIBIT 12-5 Basic Suggestions to Minimize Toxicity in the Workplace, Home, and Community Environments

· Remove, if possible, the source of any toxic materials:

Acids

Cleaning agents.

Dyes

Glues

Insecticides

Paints

Solvents

· Use an air purification system in the home, if materials cannot be removed.

· Wear protective clothing and/or breathing apparatus when using any toxic materials.

· Replace furnace and air conditioning filters in the home on a regular basis.

· Eat fresh, wholesome foods, including fruits, vegetables, grains.

· Avoid using pesticides and herbicides.

· Avoid smoking cigarettes.

Summary

Internal and external environments affect the health of the immune system. The accumulation of toxins can weaken the immune system and can cause a wide range of dysfunctions of the body and mind. In normal daily life, exposure to heavy metals, parasites, pesticides, radiation, and geopathic stress can lead to toxicity and cause serious health consequences. It is important to identify symptoms associated with toxicity and implement measures to reduce it. The approaches to reduce or prevent the accumulation of toxins in the body include good basic health practices, relaxation techniques, deep tissue massage, sauna, skin brushing, consumption of nutritional supplements, and detoxification. Because exposure to toxins is a reality of life for the average person, active steps must be taken to prevent exposure and strengthen the body's ability to resist the ill effects of toxins.

References

1. U.S. Department of Labor, Occupational Safety and Health Administration. (2008). Heavy Metals. Retrieved August 5, 2008 from http://www.osha.gov/SLTC/metalsheavy/index.html
2. Becaria, A., Campbell, A., & Bondy, S. C. (2002). Aluminum as a toxicant. *Toxicology and Industrial Health*, 18:309–320.

3. Environmental Protection Agency. (2008). *Lead in Drinking Water*. Retrieved from http://www
    .epa.gov/OGWDW/lead/basicinformation.html
4. Binns, H. J., Campbell, C., & Brown, M. J., for the Advisory Committee on Childhood Lead Poi-
    soning. (2007). Interpreting and managing blood lead levels of less than 10 _g/dL in children
    and reducing childhood exposure to lead: recommendations of the Centers for Disease Con-
    trol and Prevention Advisory Committee on Childhood Lead Poisoning Prevention. *Pediatrics*,
    120:e1285–e1298, http://pediatrics.aappublications.org/cgi/content/abstract/120/5/e1285
5. Bellinger, D. C., Trachtenberg, F., Barregard, L., Tavares, M., Cernichiari, E., Daniel, D., & McKin-
    lay, S. (2006). Neuropsychological and renal effects of dental amalgam in children: a random-
    ized clinical trial. *JAMA, 295*(15):1775–1783.

Suggested Readings

Asante-Duah, K. (2002). *Public Health Risk Assessment for Human Exposure to Chemicals*. Norwell, MA: Kluw-
    er Academic Press.
Ayres, J., Maynard, R. L., & Richards, R. (2006). *Air Pollution and Health. Academic Press*. Burlington, MA:
    Elsevier.
Bennett, P. (2001). *7-Day Detox Miracle*. Rocklin, CA: Prima Publishing.
Fitzgerald, P. (2001). *The Detox Solution*. Santa Monica, CA: Illumination Press.
Krohn, J., & Taylor, F. (2002). *Natural Detoxification* (2nd ed). Point Roberts, WA: Hartley and Marks
    Publishers.
Landner, L., & Reuther, R. (2004). *Metals in Society and in the Environment: A Critical Review of Current Knowl-
    edge on Fluxes, Speciation, Bioavailability and Risk for Adverse Effects of Nickel and Zinc*. Norwell, MA:
    Kluwer Academic Press.
Rana, S. V. S. (2006). *Environmental Pollution: Health and Toxicology*. Oxford, UK: Alpha Science.
Slaga, T. (2003). *The Detox Revolution*. New York: Contemporary Books/McGraw Hill Co.

Chapter 13

Promoting a Healing Environment

OBJECTIVES

This chapter should enable you to

· Explain *electromagnetic field*

· Describe *chakras*

· Describe energy associated with different colors

· List five factors that can influence the vibrational fields

Life is a perpetual cycle as revealed in the constant changes that occur in nature: the changing tides, the seasons, the weather patterns, and the circadian rhythm of day and night followed by the final cycle of life and death. Being part of nature, all human beings are influenced by energy cycles within the physical body as well as the vibrational or universal body that corresponds to the electromagnetic field. The electromagnetic field is multidimensional and ranges from radio waves to gamma waves. The visible spectrum of the electromagnetic field ranges from infrared to ultraviolet.

KEY POINT

During the 20th century, theorists such as Albert Einstein and Martha Rogers emerged with scientific theories that revealed man as an energy being. These theories challenged man's relationship with nature and the universe.

The electromagnetic field is referred to as the vibrational field and an individual's energy body as the vibrational body. The field that surrounds the dense physical body is known by the scientific term *electromagnetic* or *bioenergy field*. This field is depicted by ancient Christian artisans who showed the presence of a light or halo emanating from the head or crown of religious men and women. The vibrational field is comprised of at least seven layers that correspond to the physical, intellectual, and spiritual components of the visible body. Thus, both positive and negative external stimuli can have a profound impact on the body, mind, and spirit of an individual.

KEY POINT

People are more than skin and bones, thoughts and feelings. They are spectacular vibrational beings who resonate with the full-spectrum rays of the sun.

The vibrational field is hypothesized to be made of seven major *chakras*. A chakra (coming from the Sanskrit for *wheel of light*) is a spinning wheel or energy vortex that acts as a vibrational transformer within the field that extends outside the body. Although the chakra energy system is just now gaining recognition in the United States, ancient Indian Yogi literature described chakras approximately 5000 years ago.

The vibrational body is in part also comprised of seven major chakras, each of which connects with a nerve plexus, endocrine gland, and specific physiology and anatomy within a specific area of the body. The first five chakras extend from the base of the spinal column to the cervical spine, the sixth chakra to the pituitary gland, and the seventh chakra to the pineal gland. The seven major chakras resonate with the full spectrum rays from red to violet. (For a fuller discussion of chakras, see Chapter 20.)

Each chakra resonates with a musical note, as well as the sequence of the seven colors in the rainbow from infrared to ultraviolet. The chakra energy system energetically connects with the associated endocrine glands, nerve plexus, and anatomy and physiology at the individual points of origin. For example, the fourth chakra—the heart chakra—is located mid-chest and corresponds to the thymus gland, cardiac nerve plexus, heart, and lungs.

KEY POINT

The environment consists of the objects, conditions, and situations that surround us.

Sunlight

Sunlight provides a complement of the full-spectrum rays that correlate with the vibration of the seven major chakras. Although artificial light does allow us to partake in life after dark, artificial light does not resonate with the colors of the chakras. A means to correct inadequate natural sunlight or poor artificial lighting is the use of a full-spectrum light bulb in primary rooms. These are not essential in every light source.

KEY POINT

Seasonal affective disorder is a severe form of winter depression. It is characterized by lethargy, boredom, lack of joy, hopelessness, increased sleeping, and overeating. The primary factor responsible for this is the lack of natural sunlight. Natural sunlight affects the pineal gland (seventh chakra) to reduce its release of melatonin, which controls the circadian rhythm of the sleep–wake cycle. Although artificial light allows us to partake in life after dark, it does not resonate with the colors of the chakras.

Color

Color is a vibration that resonates with the chakra energy system, and it can influence the sense of well-being. The vibration flows in accordance with the full spectrum of colors of the rainbow: red, orange, yellow, green, blue, indigo, and violet. Various colors are associated with different types of energy.

Violet: spiritual energy connected to universal power and healing

Indigo: a blend of red and violet, stimulates intuition or the third eye

Blue: invokes a sense of calm

Green: a healing quality, the color of nature that supports the heart chakra

Yellow: associated with solar energy, power, and intellect

Orange: a nurturing energy related to creation, sunrise, and sunset

Red: invigorating life force in small amounts and can be energetically overwhelming with large or continual exposure

It is useful for people to determine their favorite color. After the favorite color has been identified, people should determine how much this color appears in their personal environments. It is important that the favorite color be in the immediate environment either as an accent or as a primary color. With some planning, the color can be incorporated into the environment while respecting others who share the same space. For example, a bowl of fresh oranges could be sufficient to incorporate a favorite color of orange into an area rather than painting an entire room that color. Fresh flowers, plants, fruit bowls, pillows, jewelry, and clothing of the favorite color are useful vibrational remedies that can be incorporated into daily life. People also may want to pay attention to their life's circumstances to see whether their favorite color changes as result of their experiences.

KEY POINT

Color Therapy's Struggle for Acceptance
The history of color therapy dates from 1550 BC when Egyptian priests left papyrus manuscripts showing their use of color science in their healing temples. A renewed interest in color therapy developed over the past two centuries, but was met with skepticism. For example, in 1878, Edwin Babbitt wrote a book that is referred to as the *Materia Medica* for color therapy or chromotherapy, yet during his lifetime, his thoughts and views were equally praised and criticized by his peers.[1] In the early part of the 20th century, Dinshah Ghadiali developed *spectro chrome tonation*, which was a system of attuned color waves that struggled for 40 years to gain acceptance from the American Medical Association. Roland Hunt promoted the meditative approach of color breathing and color visualization in his 1971 book, *The Seven Keys to Color Healing*;[2] however, this had little impact in mainstream healthcare circles.

Clutter

Clutter is a major stress factor that potentially irritates the nervous system. It not only disturbs the visual field, but the vibrational field as well. This is due to the fact that the vibrational field exists beyond the skin; therefore, clutter in a space can cause a restriction of that field.

Vibrational remedies for clutter begin with the simple act of examining the environment with a critical eye. People can be challenged to consider how they would like their homes to look if a special guest was visiting. They can be encouraged to begin the habit of not bringing a new item into their homes without discarding or giving away something in return. Reorganizing living space and donating unnecessary belongings can be beneficial, as can recycling (which not only reduces clutter, but helps to protect the earth). In addition to the reward of a more harmonious environment, people most likely will discover more floor space to use for relaxing or exercising.

Sound

REFLECTION

Try closing your eyes and noticing the sounds in your immediate environment. List three pleasant sounds, for example, the voices of loved ones, sounds of nature, even the absence of sound (peace and quiet). Now, list all of the negative sounds in your home or office: unpleasant verbal interactions, loud music, machinery, persistent phone ringing, household appliances, and so forth. Be aware that noise pollution can disturb the nervous system, creating an increase in stress levels. Compare your lists and try to make adjustments to reduce auditory overload and enhance positive aspects of sound in your environment.

The link between music and health is ancient and elemental. Music therapy influences the chakra energy system according to vibration and tone. The natural rhythm of the ocean, raindrops, wind-ruffled leaves, and birds chirping universally promote relaxation. Manmade music dates to the ancient cultures and mythology. Apollo, known as the god of medicine, also was the god of music. Drumming correlates to the human heartbeat. New Age music with synthesizers and string instruments connects with the higher vibrations of the chakra energy system. Today, classical music is incorporated into surgical suites, dentists' offices, and hospice facilities as a holistic, stress-reducing measure.

KEY POINT

The vibrational body can be soothed through the sound of a water fountain. People can create their own fountains with a fish tank, water pump, deep pottery bowl, and imagination.

Scents

The vibrational body adapts to most situations over time. The sense of smell is an ideal example of this. Normally, the sense of smell is keen when a scent or odor is first detected, but it then becomes less acute with continued exposure. This can create a problem in that toxic substances can permeate living areas without detection. Toxic chemicals found in the home or workplace can lead to a host of symptoms, such as headaches, nasal stuffiness, and shortness of breath related to chemical sensitivity.

KEY POINT

Radon is an inert radioactive gas that is the natural radioactive decay of radium and uranium found in the soil. Excessive levels of radon have been linked to an increased lung cancer risk. (There is a very high incidence of lung cancer in uranium miners.) Many factors determine the amount of radon that escapes from the soil to enter a house: weather, soil porosity, soil moisture, granite, and ledge. The incidence of radon is greater from water supplied from a well versus city water. (Call the EPA hotline to learn more about this problem at 1-800-SOS-RADON.)

Aromatherapy is a holistic approach that uses the essential oils extracted from plants, flowers, resins, and roots for therapeutic effects. It has an important role in promoting a healing environment (see Chapter 23).

To promote a healthy sense of smell, people should use all-natural cleaning agents and scents. It is important for people to learn to be wise consumers by reading labels looking for toxins in all products that contain artificial chemicals. Less is better when aromatics are used in the home.

KEY POINT

The basic ingredients for natural cleaning agents are white vinegar and baking soda. Essential oils such as eucalyptus, lemon, lavender, and tea tree can be added to these agents to offer antibacterial and antiviral effects.

Feng Shui

Feng shui, which grew out of Chinese astrology, is the Chinese art of arranging the environment to affect a person's internal state positively. It offers ways to align pieces of furniture that are said to promote better health, prosperity, and overall well-being. The attributes of the five elements—water, wood, fire, earth, and metal—are considered in planning an environment that is best suited for an individual.

Flavors

Food preparation is one of the greatest expressions of love. Love and caring are especially evident when an effort is made to maintain the integrity, quality, and nutritional value of all the foods that are served. Good old-fashioned home cooking can do wonders to restore the body, mind, and spirit.

A rainbow diet satisfies nutritional needs as well as the vibration of the seven chakras. To follow a rainbow diet, people need to eat as many colors in natural foods (fruits and vegetables) as there are in the rainbow. Examples of this could include red apples, orange squash, yellow lemons, green broccoli, blueberries, indigo eggplant, and purple potatoes. The rainbow diet also provides a variety of flavors, which enhances food consumption.

Touch

Touch is imperative in the development of a healthy life; nevertheless, the advent of technology has contributed to an era of touch deprivation. The ease of computer communications reduces personal interactions, such as a friendly handshake or a hearty hug. Studies have revealed that babies in hospitals or orphanages who were not picked up or nurtured suffered from a potentially life-threatening syndrome, "failure to thrive."

> **REFLECTION**
>
> Consider the amount of touch in your own life and how you can increase opportunities for touch, such as classic hugs and handshakes.

A mere touch on the hand with the intention to send healing love to someone can make a world of difference. Pets provide opportunities to touch and be touched in return. The value of touch is vital to life enhancement.

Intuition or higher sense perception is accessible to every one. It is that small inner voice—a knowing without knowing how or why—that nudges you along to pay attention to positive and negative aspects of daily life. Pay attention to caustic or harmful situations in your environment. Invite your intuitive thoughts to surface regularly as a barometer of your personal healing environment.

Summary

The body is more than physical substance. An electromagnetic field that offers energy to promote health surrounds the body. It is theorized that the body also has a vibrational field made of seven chakras, which are spinning wheels of energy. Each chakra resonates with a musical tone and represents colors in the rainbow from infrared to ultraviolet. Various colors are associated with different types of energy. The vibrational fields are influenced by color, clutter, sound, scents, flavors, and touch. People can influence their health and well-being by selecting colors that promote the desired feeling, reducing clutter, controlling noise, selecting music that is soothing, using scents therapeutically, and increasing touch contact with other people and pets. People need to develop sensitivity to the reality that positive and negative external stimuli can have a profound impact on the body, mind, and spirit.

References

1. Babbitt, E. (1942). *The Principles of Light and Color*. Whitefish, MT: Kessinger Publishing.
2. Hunt, R. (1971). *The Seven Keys to Color Therapy*. San Francisco: Harper & Row Publishers.

Suggested Readings

Bassano, M. (1992). *Healing with Music and Color*. New York: Samuel Weiser, Inc.

Cass, H. (2001). Update on seasonal affective disorder: light therapy and herbs relieve many symptoms. *Alternative and Complementary Therapies, 7*(1):5–7.

Demarco, A., and Clarke, N. (2001). An interview with Alison Demarco and Nichol Clarke: light and colour therapy explained. *Complementary Therapies in Nurse Midwifery, 7*(2):95–103.

Gardner-Gordon, J. (2006). *Vibrational Healing Through The Chakras: With Light, Color, Sound, Crystals, and Aromatherapy*. Berkeley, CA: Crossing Press.

Liberman, J. (2008). *Light: Medicine of the Future*. Santa Fe: Bear & Co.

Sharp, M. (2007). *Dossier of the Ascension: A Practical Guide to Chakra Activation and Kundalini Awakening*. Canada: Avatar.

Wong, E. (2001). *A Master Course in Feng Shui*. Boston: Shambhala Press.

Chapter 14

The Power of Touch

OBJECTIVES

This chapter should enable you to

- Describe the way touch has been used for healing throughout history
- Describe at least five touch therapies
- Discuss factors that promote healing benefits from touch
- Describe three techniques that can be used to become self-aware and have a centered heart while practicing touch

There is a mysterious healing power in touch that is beyond words and beyond our ideas about it.

AILEEN CROW

Touch . . . something we are all born to receive and to give to others. As you came into the world, you felt the touch of hands welcoming you, be it from a midwife, doctor, mother, or father. That touch was a very important one, providing you with an initial sense of safety, security, and love. As you were cradled in your mother's arms, the sense of security and love grew. You began learning the power of touch.

Touch is important in every aspect of life. It helps define a person—in his or her family and in society. All races, cultures, and religions have spoken and unspoken rules regarding touch. People learn to know when touch is and is not appropriate, to differentiate types of touch, and to evaluate whether a touch was good or bad.

In the Beginning, There Was Touch

Since the beginning of time, touch has had an important part in healing and survival. Almost instinctively, people physically reach out to those in pain, those who are suffering, those who are injured or sick, and those they love. Touch provides a soothing comfort and security.

Before the era of modern medicine as we know it, touch was a basic therapy used to compress a wound to stop it from bleeding, to caress the dying, and to welcome the newborn. Although other components of healing grew throughout time, touch remains constant.

Ancient Societies

Ancient carvings and pictures have been found throughout the world that show touch as a part of healing. In Egypt, rock carvings show hands-on healing for illness. All the ancient societies—Indian, Egyptian, Greek, Chinese, and Hebrew—used touch as part of the healing provided to their people.[1]

The Egyptians learned much of their healing techniques from the Yogis. The Greeks, in turn, learned from the Egyptians and the Indians. In ancient Athens, Aristophanes details the use of laying on of hands to heal blindness in a man and infertility in a woman.[2] In addition, the Greek priests used their hands to heal as did the physicians. As each society learned from the other, new healing modalities were added.

Native American Indians also used touch, with direct and nondirect body contact, as a method of healing. In nondirect body contact, healers hold their hands about 6 inches above the body or on opposite sides of the area needing healing. They incorporate ritual, such as cleansing the body, prayer, song, and dance, with the touch to promote healing. The Native American Indians brought to the healing process the sense of spirituality.[3]

KEY POINT

Hands-on healing, or the laying on of hands, can be found in all major religions.

Religious Stronghold

Accounts of the laying on of hands for healing can be seen in both the old and new Judeo-Christian texts. For centuries, average people have been using this type of healing with their families, friends, and others in their community. Unfortunately, the works of Plato in the early 2nd century helped stir the thinking of separating the spirit from the body. As this common belief took hold, the church also followed in its thinking of the spirit and body as separate. Touch healing came under the domain of the religious leaders or the political leaders of that particular society. Because the political leaders had such a strong association with religion, it was natural for them to assume the same or better position of authority than the religious leaders.[4]

There are many references to hands-on healing by religious and political figures. Ancient Druid priests were said to breathe on body parts and touch certain body areas in conjunction with prayer and ritual. St. Patrick helped to heal the blind, and St. Bernard healed the deaf and lame. Emperor Vespasian, Emperor Hadrian, and King Olaf were also said to have the ability to heal by touch. In fact, some of the early kings in England and France performed touch healings, which became known as the "King's touch."[5]

This power of hands-on healing began to lay solely with the priests and monarchs. Touch for healing soon began to disappear among the lay people. Unfortunately, those lay persons who continued to do hands-on healing were often labeled as pretenders to the throne or witches. Women often were targeted as witches because they made up the majority of the healers.

KEY POINT

The power of healing by women held religious, political, and sexual threats to both the ruling and religious states. From some religious viewpoints, women were considered evil because of their association with sex, and thus, it was not much of a stretch for women to be suspected of practicing witchcraft when they demonstrated their healing powers. Politically, women were viewed to be organized and hold certain power because they were the healers in their communities. By eliminating female healers, the ruling class created chaos and gained control. Sadly, it is estimated that millions of women and girls were executed in the Middle Ages under the guise of witchcraft.[6]

Science and Medicine

Medicine began with the priests and philosophers of early Egyptian and Greek thinking. Over the centuries, medicine became the domain of men and women were excluded from the profession. As medical science developed, touch as a healing act became viewed as within the domain of the church or monarchy.

Medicine considered touch to be within the realm of superstition rather than something with any scientific basis for healing. There was no hard proof that touch produced any therapeutic results; therefore, touching of patients was not needed other than that involved in performing a task. As the Age of Science developed, healing techniques and medicine became empirically based (proved by experiments). It was believed that if something could not be proved by science it did not or could not work and had to be superstition or sorcery. Touch as a healing tool could not be proved. This same thinking continued into the 20th century and only recently has gained new awareness within the medical community.

We Have Come Full Circle

With the massive amount of information available in the last several years, new knowledge has been gained about old methods of healing. With the world becoming smaller because of the mingling of cultures, computer networks, and advances in education, the old is being rediscovered. As more people turn to complementary and alternative therapies, mainstream medicine is forced to acknowledge the power of touch in healing.

The US government, through the National Institute of Health's National Center for Complementary and Alternative Medicine, is conducting research on many types of healing. One aspect of healing they are examining is the power of touch to heal. Among the touch therapies they recognize are healing touch, therapeutic touch, and massage. In addition, a significant number of schools of medicine and nursing incorporate complementary therapies as part of their educational programs.

Will Science Prove It Works?

Research indicates that touch may be so much more than the physical contact between individuals. Nursing has led the way in this research with the earliest studies from the 1970s. Dr. Delores Krieger, a nurse scientist and professor at New York University, began studying touch as therapy with the help of Dora Kunz and Oskar Estebany. Kunz was not someone who would be considered a healthcare provider based on the standards of having a license to heal someone. Rather, she was born with the ability to perceive energy around living things and describe them as accurately as a medical reference book.

Estebany was a retired colonel in the Hungarian Calvary who found he could heal animals. He was able to heal his own horse by spending the night in his stable, stroking and caressing the animal, talking to it and praying over it. By the next day, the horse was better. Soon people brought other sick animals for him to heal and then children. He became known in his country as a hands-on healer. He decided to offer his services for research and moved to Canada where he met and joined Dora Kunz.

Dr. Krieger met the two of them and decided to do research after watching them in a healing session. She observed Estebany laying hands on people wherever he sensed they were needed. He would mostly sit in silence during the 20–25-minute sessions. Kunz would observe him and redirect him to another area if she perceived another area needing treatment. Dr. Krieger found that most people reported being relaxed and that most felt better. He treated those with emphysema, brain tumors, rheumatoid arthritis, and congestive heart disease.[7]

Estebany did not think hands-on healing could be taught to other people but that it was a gift that one has. Kunz disagreed and decided to begin workshops to teach people how to do hands-on healing. Dr. Krieger joined her in these workshops and learned how to do hands-on healing, too. Together they developed therapeutic touch and began an interesting trend in research and healing. As the research developed and the outcomes began to show significant responses, the power of touch was revealed. In the past 20 years, therapeutic touch has been offered in classes and workshops in more than 80 colleges and universities in the United States and over 70 countries worldwide.

KEY POINT

Therapeutic touch is based on the principle that people are energy fields who can transfer energy to one another to promote healing. The practitioner's hands do not directly touch the client, but are held several inches above the body surface within the energy field and positioned in purposeful ways. A core element of therapeutic touch is the mindset or intent of the practitioner to help.

Another method of hands-on healing called *healing touch* was developed by nurse Janet Mentgen. This modality was inspired in part from therapeutic touch, the work of Brugh Joy, and the energy and philosophical concepts were from Rosalyn Bruyere and Barbara Brennan. It began as a pilot project at the University of Tennessee and in Gainesville, Florida in 1989. By 1990, it became a certificate program with certification beginning in 1993. This multilevel program combines healing techniques from various healers throughout the world.

KEY POINT

Healing touch is an energy-based therapy, which assists in healing the body–emotion–mind–spirit component of the self.

Healing touch is done through a centered heart, bringing to it a spiritual aspect. There is no affiliation with any one religious belief, and it can be used by those of any religion. It complements traditional healing through modern medicine and psychotherapy, but it is not used as a substitute for them. Many hospitals are now incorporating healing touch as part of patient services through specific areas within the hospital, and the use of healing touch is being studied in people with cancer, pain, depression, HIV, cardiac problems, and diabetes.

Another form of hands-on healing is *Reiki*. This Japanese-derived therapy means *universal life energy*. Reiki was developed by Dr. Mikao Usui, a Christian minister, in the middle of the 19th century. It is comprised of laying hands on the body or leaving them above the body and channeling energy to the recipient.

KEY POINT

Reiki is a form of healing in which the Reiki master channels energy to another individual.

Reiki is learned through a series of intensive sessions whereby a Reiki master passes on the knowledge to others by way of *attunements*. These attunements permit the new practitioner to be able to perform healings by touch. There is no formal certification process in the Usui system of Reiki. A student is deemed competent when a Reiki master decides so.

There are additional kinds of hands-on healing, with more being developed all of the time. Examples of others include craniosacral therapy, polarity, chakra balancing, acupressure, and shiatzu. Some involve tissue or muscle manipulation, such as neuromuscular release, Rolfing, Trager, massage therapy, and reflexology (see Exhibit 14-1). Although

---

EXHIBIT 14-1 Types of Touch Therapy and Purposes

Acupressure: Used to stimulate the body's natural self-healing ability and to allow chi to flow, the life energy of the body. The hands apply pressure to specific acupoints on the body similar to acupuncture.

Craniosacral therapy: Started in the early 1900s by Dr. William Sutherland, an osteopathic physician. He determined that the skull bones move under direct pressure. By working the skull, spine, and sacrum with gentle compression, the therapist aligns the bones and stretches underlying tissue to create balance and allow the spinal fluid to flow freely. This helps the body self-adjust.

Polarity: Created by Randolph Stone, polarity combines pressure-point therapy, diet, exercise, and self-awareness. It is based on the body having positive and negative charges. By varying hand pressure and rocking movements, the energy can be rebalanced.

Chakra balancing: An energy-based modality using the hands to balance the energy centers, or chakras, of the body.

Neuromuscular release: The goal is to assist the person in letting go by moving the limbs into and away from the body. It helps with circulation and emotional release.

Rolfing: By manipulation of muscle and connective tissue in a systematic way, the therapist helps the body readjust structurally to allow proper alignment of body segments.

Trager: Rhythmic rocking of limbs or whole body to aid in relaxing of muscles. This promotes optimal flow of blood, lymph fluid, nerve impulses, and energy.

Massage: Various types of light touch, percussion, and deep-tissue pressure by hands to assist in muscle relaxation, improved blood and lymph flow, and release of helpful chemicals naturally occurring in the body, such as endorphins.

Reflexology: By applying pressure to specific points on the body, energy movement to corresponding parts of the body are activated to clear and restore normal functioning. It can be done on the feet, hands, or ears.

they all have a slightly different belief or philosophy, they share the common denominator of touch.

Energy as a Component of Touch

There is considerable discussion today about *energy*. People state, "I don't have any energy today," "I feel energized," or " I have a lot of energy." You may have experienced these feelings and know that there is a difference between having high and low energy. After listening to an uplifting speech and hearing the thunderous applause, one may say the room was "energized" or "electrified." What is this energy that we are talking about?

REFLECTION

Do you have sensitivity to your body's energy? Are there particular experiences or people that seem to energize you and others that drain your energy?

The terms for energy date back to the older traditions of ancient cultures. Every society had a term for the life force. For some cultures, caring for this energy influenced health and wellness; by blocking or disrupting energy, disease or death could result. Other societies merely referred to it in reference to religious or spiritual beliefs. For examples of these terms, see Exhibit 14-2.

EXHIBIT 14-2   Cultural Names for Energy

Culture	Energy name
Aborigine	Arunquiltha
Ancient Egypt	Ankh
Ancient Greece	Pneuma
China	Chi (Qi)
General usage	Life force
India	Prana
Japan	Ki
Polynesia	Mana
United States	Bioenergy, biomagnetism, subtle energy

The Role of Chi

The Chinese culture has used the idea of energy for thousands of years through the philosophy of *chi (qi)*, or life force, which is an energetic substance that flows from the environment into the body. The chi flows through the body by means of 12 pairs of meridians (energy pathways to provide life-nourishing and sustaining energy). The organs of the body are affected by the pairs of meridians. There needs to be a balance of chi flowing through each side of the paired meridian in order for balance to occur and health to be attained and/or maintained.

Science is beginning to get a better understanding of this energy, what it is, and how it functions. Some researchers have developed machinery to try to detect this energy. Although success has been limited for some, others have been more successful.

KEY POINT

Motoyama, a Japanese researcher, developed a machine to assist in the detection of meridian lines within the tissues of humans. He found that these meridians do exist and that an energy flow, he calls *ki*, travels through the body. Motoyama states that a center in the brain controls the movement of ki.[8] In addition, these meridians feed the different organ systems of the body. By using his machine, called the *AMI machine*, he has been able to detect strong correlations between meridians that have energy imbalances to organs systems, which have diseases present. His machine is being used in the research of Parkinson's disease at the Bob Hope Parkinson Research Institute in Florida.

The Energy Fields or Auras

In addition to the seven chakras (see Chapter 20 for an explanation of chakras), there exist seven layers of energy fields, or auric fields, around the body. These energy fields surround all living and nonliving matter. Science has begun to study and explain these fields over the last several years. The science of physics has done the most extensive work in explaining energy fields. Through Newtonian physics, field theory, and Einstein's theory of relativity, a better understanding of how energy works has been acquired, but it is quantum physics that has really helped explain the characteristics and behaviors of energy. Since then, many scientists have begun looking at things as a *hologram* (a multidimensional piece of something whole). The discussion of specifics is beyond this chapter; however, it is intended to show that science is now rethinking some of its early and persistent cause and effect notions.

One way energy fields have been viewed is through *Kirlian photography*, which was created in the 1940s by a Russian researcher, Semyon Kirlian. By using this form of photography, he was able to measure changes in the energy fields of living systems. He found that cancer causes significant changes in the electromagnetic field around the body. One of the best known experiments is that of the Phantom Leaf Effect, whereby a portion of a leaf was cut away and Kirlian photography done on the amputated leaf. Amazingly, the leaf still appeared whole with an energy field present in the form and space of the cutaway portion.

In other important work, a Japanese researcher named Motoyama, has developed a number of electrode devices to measure the human energy field at various distances from the body.[9] Thus, it is now possible to measure the excess or lack of energy around the body and determine a person's health status. Future technology advances may allow a body to be scanned and the beginnings of disease detected before symptoms appear in the physical body. In fact, a new CT scan is being used for this very reason to detect early onset of heart disease and cancer.

Where exactly are these fields, however? As stated previously, there are seven energy fields that are generally accepted by most energy workers. Each field corresponds to a specific chakra, for example, the first energy field with the first chakra and so on; however, the fields lay one on top of another yet do not interfere with each other's functions. These fields interconnect yet maintain their own separateness.

KEY POINT

Energy fields of the body work similar to a television. When you change channels, you get a different picture. All of the pictures do not end up on the same channel, but they do come through one television set. Likewise, when listening to a radio, you change stations to hear different music, but you still have one radio. The same idea works for the energy fields of the body.

When two people interact, their energy fields connect and they can pick up information about each other. For example, you are riding on an elevator, and a stranger gets on. You do not say anything to the person, but you feel safe and secure. At another floor, a second person gets on. Immediately you feel uncomfortable with this person even though you have not spoken to him either. What is occurring is the intermixing of energy fields, which is giving you subconscious information about these people. It has nothing to do with what they are wearing or how they look.

One of the leading causes of illness in our society is stress, yet stress is not internal. Stress originates outside the body and works its way inward through the energy fields and chakras. It is a well-known fact that long-term stress can weaken the immune system's response and cause heart attacks, high blood pressure, and depression. Of course, there are physical evidences for each of these, but the process starts long before any physical evidence is detected. How does this occur? It is thought that long-term stress causes changes in the energy fields and chakras that over time repattern themselves and begin to affect the cells of the body. Depending on the severity of the repatterning, illness and disease can occur. By addressing the stressors, one is able to fix or heal any changes made in the energy field or chakras.

Humans as Multidimensional Beings

This concept of energy fields and chakras intermixing contributes to humans being multi-dimensional. In other words, you are made up of more than just your parts. You not only contain energy, but you are energy that is constantly changing. The body uses energy to perform its functions: for nerves to stimulate muscles, the beating of the heart, lungs to exchange air, cells to digest nutrients, and the creation of an idea. There is nothing in the body that is not involved in some form of energy. When the normal energy flow is inter-rupted or destroyed, the body is unable to function to its fullest capacity, and illness, disease, and disability can develop. When all of the energy workings cease, death occurs.

Nevertheless, quantum physics has shown us that energy cannot be destroyed. Thus, when we die, it is just the physical part of ourselves that dies. The energy that aided us in our physical form transforms and is released into the environment; therefore, one does not die—the physical body is just transformed.

Touch is Powerful

With this discussion of the energy systems of the body, you can see that a touch is not just a simple physical act. Something happens human to human, human to animal, human to plant, and animal to animal when touch occurs. This exchange of energy affects not only the one receiving the touch, but also the one giving the touch.

KEY POINT

One of the most important aspects of touch is its intention.

There are neutral touches, such as tapping someone on the arm to get their attention. In addition, there are those touches out of anger that are meant to hurt someone, like a slap or kick. Then there are the loving touches of a hug or caress. The intention is what differ-entiates.

The way to obtain the power of touch for healing is through a centered heart. This is done in several ways. It occurs spontaneously for couples in love or in the love that a parent